Anthropological Papers
Museum of Anthropology, University of Michigan
No. 77

Jumano and Patarabueye
Relations at La Junta de los Rios

by
J. Charles Kelley
with a foreword by John D. Speth

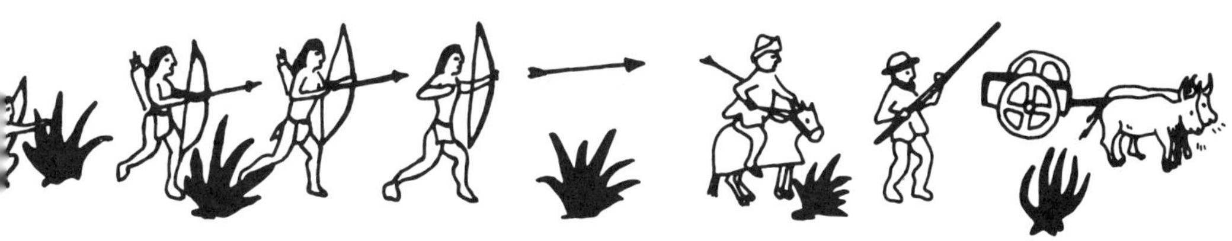

Ann Arbor, Michigan
1986

Printed in the
United States of America

ISBN 0-915703-05-X

Contents

Illustrations

FIGURES

PLATES

Preface—1986

My 1947 dissertation, published here for the first time, had its origins in a manuscript on the Jumano Indians which I wrote in 1935 during my junior year at the University of New Mexico. In the spring of 1935 this initial version was awarded the Hodge Ethnohistory Award (with a cash value of $25). Frederick Webb Hodge had established this award the previous year when the University had conferred upon him an honorary doctoral degree. It should be noted that my manuscript was the only one submitted in the competition! Discussions with Hodge that summer when he visited my field camp at Steamboat Canyon on the Navaho Reservation further stimulated my interest in the Jumanos. In 1936, I had the opportunity of visiting La Junta de los Rios and digging a stratigraphic trench in what was putatively a Jumano archaeological site.

As library and field research continued, I became increasingly aware of the Patarabueyes. Soon it became clear that the Jumanos and the Patarabueyes must be regarded as distinct groups. The documentary evidence was confirmed by excavations which Donald Lehmer and I were able to carry out in 1938–39 at the Millington site at La Junta, and by my own excavations at the Loma Alta site in 1939. Subsequently, during excavations made under my supervision in central Texas, I was able to identify archaeological proof of the Jumano presence, already established by documentary evidence. By 1947 the original 1935 manuscript had undergone more than ten revisions and I was almost ready to attempt its publication.

Meanwhile, I continued work on a dissertation topic previously approved by my Harvard committee. Early in the fall of 1947 I was advised by my department chairman at the University of Texas that under the "up-

or-out" rule a tenure committee would be appointed for me the following spring and that if I did not by that time have my Ph.D. in hand, I had no chance of approval. The chairman of my dissertation committee informed me that the degree could be awarded at mid-year if my dissertation and dissertation examination could be completed during December. Somewhat reluctantly the committee approved substitution of the existing Jumano-Patarabueye manuscript for the original approved topic, but noted that many changes would have to be made in the manuscript to convert it into approved dissertation format.

A date in December was set for the dissertation examination. Long hours of work during the fall enabled me to complete the dissertation in time for the examination, but much of it was hurriedly written and I was not able to edit the final paper until I was enroute to Boston by train. By special dispensation of the committee I was allowed to take—and pass—the dissertation examination using the uncorrected version; corrections were made thereafter. Because of the hasty preparation of the dissertation and the many corrections made in the final version, this document represents what is probably the worst dissertation ever accepted at Harvard University.

In the spring of 1948 I submitted the document to the University of Texas for possible publication. Publication was refused on the grounds that dissertations, as such, should not be published. I made no further attempt to have it published and my only final copy of it was largely destroyed by water damage when fire hoses were turned into my office when Old Main Building at Southern Illinois University, Carbondale, was destroyed by fire. Accordingly, I was quite pleased when Dr. John D. Speth suggested that he could probably arrange for its publication in the Anthropology Papers of the University of Michigan Museum of Anthropology.

I agreed with Dr. Speth that the dissertation should be published as is, with no attempt to update it. I had not participated actively in archaeological research in Texas since 1950, when I became Director of the University Museum at Southern Illinois University, Carbondale. Too much time would be required for any major revision, and my own advanced age and state of health made it improbable that a revised version would ever be completed. Even preparing the original dissertation for publication has proved difficult. The text could be reproduced from a Xerox copy of the original dissertation, but copies of the photographic plates and line drawings were not usable. Luckily most of the original illustrations had been preserved in my files, but considerable deterioration had occurred over the intervening 38 years. Some illustrations could be partially restored; others had to be used as they were.

The question arises as to the advisability of publishing without revision a manuscript prepared in 1947. The principal justification is that no other researcher has covered the same ground in the intervening period. Indeed, more than one researcher has continued to confuse the Jumanos and the Patarabueyes. In effect, the Jumanos disappeared as a group by A.D. 1700, but references to agricultural villages at La Junta, identified as Patarabueye in this dissertation, appear frequently in the historic documents throughout the eighteenth century. Neither Jumano nor Patarabueye archaeology can be understood without utilization of this distinction.

The ethnohistory of the Jumanos as traced in this document remains essentially correct and complete. Very few additional references to the group have been discovered in other sources in the intervening 38 years and no scholar has duplicated this study. On the other hand, an enormous mass of new data has been accumulated by archaeological research in Texas during this period and all conclusions regarding Jumano archaeology in this document are subject to revision.

Similarly, the ethnohistory of the Patarabueyes as presented here remains essentially correct, but much new data have appeared and one major change regarding the location of the La Junta villages is required. Not until after this dissertation was written did I obtain access to the vitally important diaries of the La Junta *entradas* of Joseph de Idoiaga, Pedro de Rabago y Teran, and Fermin de Vidaurre in 1746–1748. Not only do these accounts add considerable new data regarding the Patarabueyes, they also clarify the locations of the La Junta pueblos and expose an error which I made in this dissertation. In it I locate the La Junta pueblo of Nuestra Señora de Guadalupe on the Texas bank of the joined rivers at the archaeological site of Shafter 7:1, the Millington site. But the 1746–1748 documents clearly identify the present site of Ojinaga, Chihuahua, as the location of Guadalupe, and place the pueblo of San Cristobál at the Millington site location. These documents also enable a more precise location of other La Junta pueblos and emphasize strongly the continued existence of the Patarabueye villages long after the Jumanos have disappeared from the local scene. I have corrected these errors and added the new data from the 1746–1748 *entradas* in a paper published in 1952–1953.

Patarabueye archaeology remains as described in this dissertation. Surprisingly, no substantial excavations have been made in the Patarabueye pueblo archaeological sites of the La Junta area since the termination of my own field work there. This dissertation hence remains essentially the primary source for our knowledge of the La Junta pueblos, justification in itself for its publication. Unfortunately, there has been considerable vandalism of these sites and despite the strenuous efforts of Robert Mallouf, Texas State Archaeologist (aided by Enrique Madrid of Redford, Texas), to preserve these sites. The largest of them all, the Millington site, is now endangered by real estate development in Presidio, Texas. It is to be hoped that in this generation archaeologists equipped with techniques, methods, and instrumentation not available to us 38 years ago will again excavate in the important La Junta sites. Then, and not until then, will it be possible to further clarify Patarabueye archaeology and correct errors that I must certainly have made in my own interpretations.

Belatedly, I wish to express very real gratitude to the members of my dissertation committee at Harvard University: Clyde Kluckhohn (chairman), J. O. Brew, Donald Scott, Kirk Bryan, and Alfred Kidder II. They were tolerant of my many small errors because they believed the total dissertation was adequate. My debt of gratitude is especially strong to the late Clyde Kluckhohn who was for many years my anthropological mentor. Without his aid and encouragement I would not have been able to attend Harvard, and in all probability would not have continued my graduate studies to the doctorate.

In regard to the present publication I am deeply grateful to John D. Speth, and to Ms. Sally Horvath, Editor, not only for resurrecting this paper, but also for making a very serious attempt to turn it into a respectable monograph. I also wish to thank my wife, Ellen Abbott Kelley, for her perseverance in searching through a nearly endless accumulation of ancient files in order to retrieve most of the original illustrations for the monograph.

J. Charles Kelley
Fort Davis, Texas
1986

References

Idoiaga, Joseph de
1746–1747 Quaderno que comienze con la Carta Orden del Exmó. Señor Virrey, Gouernador y Capitan General de estos Reynos, de resulta de mi Consulta y Diligencias.... Archivo General de Indias, Audiencia de Mexico, 89–2–3; Dunn Transcripts, 1746–47, Archives Collection, University of Texas. Pages 44/27–52/32 (cf. p. 34/252–253).

Kelley, J. Charles
1952, *1953* The Historic Indian Pueblos of La Junta de los Rios. Parts 1 and 2. *New Mexico Historical Review*, 27(4):257–95 and 28(1):21–51.

Teran, Pedro de Rabago y
1747 Diario de la Campana executada por el Governor de Coahuila Don Pedro de Rabago y Teran en el ano de 1747.... Mexico, Archivo General de la Nacion. Historia, Vol. 52, Expediente No. 6. Hackett Transcripts, Archives Collection, University of Texas.

Vidaurre, Fermin de
1747–1748 Derrotero, Diario, y Autos Echos por el capn del Rl Presidio de Santiago de Mapimi D. Fermin de Vidaurre.... Mexico, Archivo General de la Nacion. Historia, Vol. 53, Expediente No. 8. Hackett Transcripts, Archives Collection, University of Texas.

Preface—1947

I became interested in the Jumano problem over ten years ago. The first draft of the present monograph was written in 1936. Dr. France V. Scholes, who was at that time preparing his own paper on the Jumanos for publication, kindly read and criticized my original manuscript. As a result of his criticisms, I decided that my paper was inadequate. Since that time I have continued my research on the Jumanos, both in the library and in the field. At the present time I believe that the possibilities of library research have been almost exhausted, until new documentary evidence is found in the archives.

The archaeological approach to the Jumano problem is only in its initial stage, however. Much work remains to be done in Texas, both reconnaissance and excavation, in the vital areas of the Concho River and the small tributaries of the Pecos River, such as Toyah and Comanche creeks, purportedly strongholds of the Jumanos. Continuation of detailed archaeological studies in the La Junta area should also add much to the eventual solution of the problem.

The trail of the Jumanos led directly to the Patarabueyes. Perhaps the principal contribution that this paper makes is the establishment of the separate identity of the Patarabueyes. Furthermore, the relations of the Jumanos and the Patarabueyes suggest the explanation for many of the observed phenomena of the growth of aboriginal culture in Texas. Here we have demonstrated not only the diffusion of ideas but the means whereby the diffusion took place.

Linguistic evidence has not been considered in the preparation of this monograph. I do not have the necessary linguistic training to compile and interpret the pertinent data, and I have therefore left this task for some future worker.

Free use has been made of the valuable studies of Herbert E. Bolton. My outline of Jumano history is little better than a paraphrase of Bolton's paper on the Jumanos. Cultural details and the continuity of the Jumano group, to the exclusion of pseudo-Jumano references, have been emphasized, however, and a few references not available to Bolton, or at least not used by him, have been included. In all possible instances (and there were only a few exceptions), Bolton's documentary material has been checked from the viewpoint of this paper. In practically all instances my independent interpretations are in complete accord with Bolton's.

Scholes's valuable work has been of considerable utility in the present study, and I have profited likewise from the archaeological research of E. B. Sayles, as well as that of my colleagues Alex D. Krieger, T. N. Campbell, and Donald J. Lehmer.

I have received invaluable aid in the actual preparation of the paper from my wife, Lois Neville Kelley, who prepared many of the illustrations, aided in typing, and provided constant inspiration for the continuation of the study. Ruby Oncken has aided materially in the final preparation of the report, and my stepdaughter, Joyce Neville, has spent many midnight hours typing and retyping the manuscript. Patricia Anne McGregor did much of the final typing, and Marian Silver and Herbert C. Taylor aided in the final proofreading. I wish to express my sincere appreciation for the aid of all of these people, as well as that of many others not here named.

The present paper by no means supplies the final word on the Jumano problem. The need for further archaeological work and linguistic study has already been indicated. The Patarabueyes should, and probably will, be studied intensively in future years. Even those points that appear to be amply demonstrated in this paper should still be considered probabilities rather than facts, and hence subject to further study.

J. Charles Kelley
December 12, 1947

Foreword—1986

Along the southern and eastern peripheries of the Greater Southwest, relatively sedentary puebloan economies based on small-scale farming give way to more nomadic hunting and gathering economies, providing one of the most fascinating anthropological laboratories in North America. Preserved in the archaeological record of the periphery, and documented in innumerable Spanish archival sources, is clear evidence that the boundary between these seemingly polar economic and social entities has been anything but sharp, and that over the centuries its nature and position have shifted repeatedly and often dramatically. Thus, right here in our own backyard may be the key to a problem that has compelled anthropologists to travel to the four corners of the globe: what encourages horticulturalists and hunter-gatherers to engage at times in close, amicable exchange relations and alliances with one another, occasionally giving rise to tightly interdependent or mutualistic economic systems, and at other times to shift to strategies of avoidance, deceit, sporadic raiding, or even warfare (cf. Spielmann 1982)? Also preserved in these same sites and archives are keys to understanding the processes by which nomadic foraging economies sometimes may be completely transformed, often quite suddenly, into village farming communities, or the reverse in which farmers abandon their agrarian pursuits and become foragers.

These are mainstream issues in anthropology today. One need only look at the current debates about whether the Kalahari San have been "pristine" hunters and gatherers since the Pleistocene, or instead have oscillated back and forth between foraging and pastoralism (Schrire 1980; Wilmsen 1983). Nor is this debate unique to the San. Similar discussions are going on today concerning the Ituri Pygmies. For many years our view of the Pygmies was essentially the picture painted by Colin Turnbull (1961) of an enduring and completely self-contained way of life intimately tied to the resources of a beneficent tropical forest. More recent work has turned this view on its head, suggesting instead that the Pygmies are specialized providers of meat, hides, and occasional labor for neighboring Bantu villagers. Some have even gone so far as to argue that the Pygmies could not have survived in the Ituri Forest without access to the reliable carbohydrates produced by the farmers (Bahuchet and Guillaume 1982; Harako 1976; Bailey and Peacock 1986). Southeast Asian hunter-gatherers, such as the Agta, Batak, and many others, also are the focus of similar discussions (Peterson 1978; Eder 1978). Where anthropologists once viewed hunter-gatherers and farmers as discrete, separate, and virtually immutable ethnic, sociopolitical, and economic entities, we now see emerging a dramatically different view in which these seemingly disparate systems interact on a regular basis, and not infrequently transform themselves from one into the other and back again. Our understanding of pastoralist-farmer relationships has undergone very similar changes in recent years (cf. Bates and Lees 1977). Archaeologists also are keenly interested in these discussions because they concern two of the field's perennial questions—the emergence of sedentism and the origins of agriculture.

Of vital importance to the development and evaluation of these newly emerging ideas are detailed data on patterns of economic and social interaction that span long periods of time. But adequate time depth often is not available. Thus, most ethnographic studies span only a few months to, at best, a few years, and few such studies predate the latter half of the nineteenth century. To expand the temporal window, ethnologists are turning more and more to archaeologists and ethnohistorians for help. This is clearly exemplified by recent work on the San. Early European accounts from southern Africa are being scoured for insights into the patterns of interaction between the San and pastoralists. These insights are being supported and fleshed out by archaeological data which document the timing of the introduction of domestic animals into the region, and changes in their distribution and use over time. These studies are rapidly changing prior conceptions that the "pristine" hunter-gatherers of southern Africa were untouched by, and oblivious to, the pastoral populations of the region. What is emerging in place of this older view is a far more complex one, in which the degree of forager-pastoral interaction varied both in degree and form through time and over space. Thus, at times San were fulltime foragers, at other times they performed labor for the pastoralists, and at still other times they obtained sheep and became pastoralists themselves.

Unfortunately, cases such as the San, which are reasonably well documented and span a relatively long period of time, are very rare.

Therein lies the incalculable value of the case reported by J. Charles Kelley in this volume. At the junction of the Conchos River with the Rio Grande (La Junta de los Rios), near the present-day towns of Ojinaga, Chihuahua, and Presidio, Texas, are the remains of a number of pueblo-like villages, some founded as early as the thirteenth century, that were visited repeatedly by Spanish missionaries, military expeditions, and explorers. In the unusually voluminous archival records that survive, many dating back to the sixteenth century, are descriptions of highly mobile buffalo hunters—the Jumanos—who wintered each year in these villages, living side-by-side with farmers—the Patarabueyes—despite the fact that the two groups differed culturally in many respects and spoke different, perhaps even unrelated, languages. The Jumanos provided the Patarabueyes with bison meat and hides, and probably protection, in exchange for corn and other items. Each spring, the Jumanos left the La Junta villages and wandered over vast areas of central and eastern Texas, hunting buffalo, foraging wild plant foods, and trading or fighting with countless other groups, both sedentary and nomadic. The Spanish documents, painstakingly analyzed by Kelley, provide invaluable descriptions of the economic and social interactions between the Jumanos and Patarabueyes, and allow the changes in these interactions to be charted over several centuries.

But the value of Kelley's study of the Jumanos and Patarabueyes goes far beyond his detailed treatment of the archival sources. Kelley has definitively located the remains of a number of the villages described by the Spanish and, through pioneering excavations carried out in the 1930s and 1940s, he succeeded in fleshing out many critical material and organizational elements of Jumano and Patarabueye economy and society that were unclear or not mentioned in the archives.

Kelley's research, though carried out more than forty years ago, demonstrates the tremendous value of the La Junta case and provides a solid foundation for further ethnohistoric and archaeological work in the area. Unfortunately, his major study on La Junta de los Rios, presented as a doctoral dissertation at Harvard University in 1947, has remained in obscurity, and largely inaccessible, ever since.

The Museum of Anthropology of the University of Michigan is extremely pleased to be able to bring this important document out of obscurity and make it available for the first time to the profession. While parts of the study are obviously out-of-date, it contains a wealth of information, available nowhere else, whose importance far outweighs the parts that are no longer current. Above all, the study clearly demonstrates the tremendous ethnohistoric and archaeological potential of the La Junta area for contributing to our understanding of hunter-gatherer/ horticultural interaction. This makes the volume of interest not only to local specialists but also to a much broader range of scholars. We hope that publication of Kelley's dissertation will stimulate renewed interest in this fascinating region, leading to further work in the archives, and especially to additional archaeological research at La Junta, before the fragile record of the Jumanos and Patarabueyes vanishes forever.

No major substantive changes have been made in the text; it is presented here almost exactly as in the original dissertation. The only major change, largely a stylistic one, was the incorporation directly into the text of a long and somewhat cumbersome series of endnotes, leaving only a few notes at the end of the book which contain important, but supplementary, information. Several of the figures had to be touched up to make them more legible or to correct for damage that occurred many years ago in a fire at Southern Illinois University.

I would like to express my sincerest gratitude to J. Charles Kelley and Enrique R. Madrid for generously taking me on a grand tour of the La Junta area to see firsthand the marvelous archaeological record of the region. This trip convinced me that La Junta de los Rios contains one of the most important and exciting archaeological records in western North America, one that desperately deserves conservation and further research. I would also like to thank our editor, Sally Horvath, our artist, Kay Clahassey, and Charles Hastings for the superb job they have done in producing the final publication.

John D. Speth
Ann Arbor, Michigan

References

Bahuchet, Serge, and Henri Guillaume
1982 Aka-Farmer Relations in the Northwest Congo Basin. In *Politics and History in Band Societies*, edited by Eleanor Leacock and Richard Lee, pp. 189–211. New York: Cambridge University Press.

Bailey, Robert C., and Nadine R. Peacock
1986 Efe Pygmies of Northeast Zaire: Subsistence Strategies in the Ituri Forest. In *Uncertainty in the Food Supply*, edited by I. de Garine and G. A. Harrison. Cambridge: Cambridge University Press (in press).

Bates, Daniel G., and Susan H. Lees
1977 The Role of Exchange in Productive Specialization. *American Anthropologist*, 79:824–41.

Eder, James F.
1978 The Caloric Returns to Food Collecting: Disruption and Change Among the Batak of the Philippine Tropical Forest. *Human Ecology*, 6:55–69.

Harako, R.
1976 The Mbuti as Hunters: A Study of Ecological Anthropology of the Mbuti Pygmies (Zaire). *Kyoto University African Studies*, 10:37–99.

Peterson, Jean T.
1978 *The Ecology of Social Boundaries: Agta Foragers of the Philippines.* Illinois Studies in Anthropology No. 11. Urbana: University of Illinois Press.

Schrire, Carmel
1980 An Inquiry into the Evolutionary Status and Apparent Identity of San Hunter-Gatherers. *Human Ecology,* 8(1):9–32.

Spielmann, Katherine A.
1982 Inter-societal Food Acquisition Among Egalitarian Societies: An Ecological Study of Plains/Pueblo Interaction in the American Southwest. Unpublished Ph.D. dissertation. Ann Arbor: University of Michigan.

Turnbull, Colin
1961 *The Forest People: A Study of the Pygmies of the Congo.* New York: Simon and Schuster.

Wilmsen, Edwin N.
1983 The Ecology of Illusion: Anthropological Foraging in the Kalahari. *Reviews in Anthropology,* 10(1):9–20.

Jumano and Patarabueye

Introduction

In the year 1811 Father José Antonio Pichardo discussed at some length a group of Indians known to the Spaniards as the Jumanos (Jumanas, Humanas, Xumanas, etc.), and to the French as the Choumanes.[1] Beginning with Adolph Bandelier in 1890, a series of prominent scholars have considered in detail the many problems arising in regard to this same Jumano group. Following Bandelier, such scholars as Hodge in 1911, Bolton in 1911, Sauer in 1934, and Scholes and Mera in 1940 have published discussions of the Jumano Indians, either as separate papers or in connection with broader studies.

With the exception of one, the scholars noted have drawn their inspiration, in succession, from the preceding papers. Bandelier, the exception, apparently did not know of the work of Pichardo; Pichardo's treatise was prepared in Spanish between 1808 and 1812, but remained in manuscript form until translated into English and published by Hackett in 1931–34. In each of the above papers some new data have been presented, the general picture reorganized, certain conclusions reached, and usually further problems recognized. This monograph differs from previous ones in that its new information is derived from archaeological research rather than from purely historical sources. (Although Mera approached the Jumano problem from an archaeological viewpoint, strictly speaking, he applied the findings of historical research to certain archaeological problems rather than contributing archaeological data to the solution of the Jumano problem.) Archaeological discoveries of recent years have made a reexamination of the historical materials necessary, as Scholes and Mera forecast in 1940, and in reexamining them, a somewhat different set of conclusions and problems have been postulated.

In presenting a new paper on the Jumanos at this time, it seems necessary to justify the continued attention given to this comparatively little known group. Further study of the Jumano problem is important for three reasons.

First, to clarify the extremely muddled picture of protohistoric and historic cultures of Texas and northwest Mexico, references to the Jumano Indians must be separated from references to other groups erroneously called Jumanos, in particular the Patarabueyes of La Junta de los Rios.

Second, the Jumano Indians appear to be of anthropological interest and importance. They emerge in the seventeenth century, if not earlier, as ethnic links between the outposts of Southwestern and North Mexican culture on the west and Southeastern culture on the east, through the intermediate southern extension of the Plains culture. Potentially, and probably in actuality, they were *culture carriers* of the highest order. As their activities and cultural relations come to light, the key to some of the major problems of North American culture history may be revealed, as well as a mechanism of culture diffusion in general.

Third, the Patarabueye Indians are revealed as peripheral Southwesterners of respectable antiquity at La Junta. Their culture appears to be a curious admixture of Southwestern and Plains traits with perhaps a flavor of Southeastern and Mexican influence. They *may* have been influential in late prehistoric and early historic times as the cultural filter through which dilute Mexican and Southwestern (and certainly European) traits were passed eastward.

Part I

The Jumano Problem

1
History and Present Status of the Jumano Problem

Pichardo anticipated many of the conclusions of more recent scholars, although his interest in the Jumanos was purely incidental. Pichardo attempted to prove the prior discovery by Spain of east Texas. One of his arguments was that the Quiviras discovered by Coronado in 1541 were in actuality the Tejas Indians of east Texas. He used the Jumano data in connection with this apparently erroneous notion, and consequently, many of his ideas were warped by his preconceived beliefs in this regard. According to him, the Jumano Indians were the native occupants of the San Clemente River area (possibly the upper Colorado River of Texas) in west-central Texas, living to the south of the Tabayaces (Taovaya-Wichita) and west of Indians known to the Spaniards as the Jumanas, Humanas, Xumanas, Choma, and Choman, and to the French as the Chouman, or Choumanes. They were the friends and neighbors of the Tejas and the Quiviras, and of the Julimes of the Rio del Norte near La Junta, but were enemies of the Apaches. They had friendly relations with the Spaniards at La Junta, where they also received religious instruction, and with the French in south and east Texas. During the late seventeenth century they were led by an Indian named Juan Sabeata. Pichardo noted that the term Jumano was sometimes mistakenly applied to other tribes, such as the Panipiques (Pawnee?) on the Arkansas River: "They were named Panipiques, all were painted, and the Spaniards call them Jumanes." But, he continued, "are these Jumanes . . . the same ones to whose lands . . . Mendoza and others went . . . ? My belief is that in fact they are very different, and . . . if at present the Spaniards call the Panipiques Jumanes, it is because of an error arising from lack of communication with them" (Pichardo, in Hackett 1931–1934:427). Here he just missed anticipating, by almost a century and a half, Scholes's conclusion that the term "Jumano" was often applied to painted or tattooed Indians in general. Unfortunately, Pichardo's work was unwittingly ignored by later scholars, who did not immediately rediscover many of the facts that he noted.

Bandelier identified the Jumanos as a tribe of sedentary Indians of Chihuahua living along the Rio Conchos and Rio Grande, especially at La Junta, though found at times far to the east in Texas. He noted that they were found at La Junta as early as 1582 and as late as 1683, and suggested that they may have been absorbed into an Apache tribe in the eighteenth century. He felt that their linguistic classification by Orozco y Berra as a branch of the Faraones Apaches was groundless. Bandelier was puzzled by the lack of reference to Jumanos at La Junta between 1583 and 1683, and after 1715, when missions were established there again. He was also confused by the apparently contradictory statements regarding the occupants of La Junta in 1683, noting that Jumano and Julimes Indians were variously listed as living together there. He concluded that either the Jumanos and Julimes lived together at La Junta, thus anticipating one of the conclusions of this book, or that the Julimes were perhaps only a branch of the Jumanos (Bandelier 1890).

Hodge identified the Jumanos of La Junta as the "People of the Cows" described by Cabeza de Vaca in 1535, and as the Patarabueyes that Espejo found living at La Junta in 1582. He characterized them as an erratic wandering tribe of semi-agricultural Indians distinguished by the trait of tattooing, a custom which gave rise in 1598 to their alternative Spanish name, *Rayados*. He noted that the Jumanos were found in eastern New Mexico in 1598, again in 1629, and after that appeared on the plains of Texas and Kansas. He concluded that the Jumanos were identical with the Tawehash (Taovayas), a branch of the Wichitas (and, hence, linguistically of Caddoan stock), and that their final disappearance could be explained by their absorption into the Wichita tribe (Hodge 1911).

Bolton accepted the identification of the Jumanos as the "People of the Cows" and as the Patarabueyes of La Junta. He traced the history of the Jumanos in central and southwest Texas, demonstrating that the "Rio Nueces" on which they were reportedly found from 1629 to 1684 was actually the Concho River, a branch of the Colorado, near San Angelo, Texas. Tracing the activities of the Jumanos under the leadership of Juan Sabeata, he showed conclusively that the Jumanos of the Rio del Norte were the same ones found in central and southwest Texas, and the Jumanos of the Spaniards were the Chouman of the French. During this period, he noted, the Jumanos were friends and allies of the Tejas Indians and the Spaniards, and deadly enemies of the Apaches. After 1716 this was reversed: the same group came to be regarded as allies of the Apaches and enemies of the Spaniards, and after 1733 they were actually known as

Apaches. Then, in 1771, a great battle was reported in which the Jumano-Apaches, with other Apache groups, came out victorious over the Comanches and Taguaias (Taovayas). Since the Taovayas were the Wichita group identified by Hodge as the Jumanos, the remarkable picture of the two Jumano tribes at war with each other was presented. Bolton was puzzled by this apparent contradiction and left it an open question (Bolton 1911).

Sauer's consideration of the Jumanos was only a casual one; his interest lay in the distribution of languages and tribes in northwestern Mexico as a whole. Nevertheless, he contributed several important points to the solution of the Jumano problem. Following Hodge, he accepted the "People of the Cows" as Jumanos, and also subscribed to the general belief that the Jumanos and the Patarabueyes were identical. He also believed that the Jumanos and the Sumas had the same speech, basing his conclusion largely on de Vaca and Espejo, and classified both groups as of Uto-Aztecan affiliation. He concluded that the Jumanos were pushed eastward onto the plains by the spread of the Conchos Indians toward La Junta; that the Plains Jumanos were absorbed into both Caddoan and Athapascan groups; and that the Jumanos who remained at La Junta were absorbed by the Conchos. He identified the Cholomes and the Cibolas as Jumano remnants at La Junta (Sauer 1934).

The most recent contribution to the solution of the Jumano problem was that of Scholes and Mera (1940:271–89). Scholes, using the historical approach, acknowledged that the identification of the Jumanos as the Patarabueyes was a dubious one and that further investigation was required. He demonstrated that the name Jumano was applied to the Quiviras (Wichitas) because they were *rayados,* and that the name was applied in New Mexico to *rayados,* or tattooed Indians, in general. Scholes considered in minute detail the history of the "Jumano" pueblos in eastern New Mexico, identifying these as the southeastern Tompiro towns of the Pueblo culture. They were called "Jumano" towns because many of their occupants were *rayados* and because *rayados* Indians from the Plains traded there. Scholes believed that a strong Plains element might have been present in this Tompiro ethnic and cultural mixture. He also reviewed the convincing evidence that the Patarabueyes and the Sumas were of the same linguistic stock, and gave important evidence that the language of the Jumano Indians and that of the Sumas were related. He likewise cast doubt upon the existence of a separate Jumano tribe or group of tribes in view of the common application of the term Jumano to any tattooed or painted people.

Mera (Scholes and Mera 1940:291–99) discussed the archaeology of southeastern New Mexico, describing an early widespread culture characterized by rancheria-type settlements, agriculture, and brown-ware pottery. This early culture was later intruded upon and modified by the Pueblo-type culture. The southeastern Pueblo towns identified as Jumano pueblos show many non-Puebloan traits, suggesting survival of the old brown-ware culture. Since the "Jumano" pueblos were thought to have been occupied by a mixed ethnic and cultural group made up of both Jumano and Pueblo elements, the identification of the old brown-ware culture as that of the Jumanos was suggested.

The conclusions of the above writers that seem to survive in a more or less acceptable form are as follows.

1) The name Jumano, or its phonetic variants, was applied to several groups, including:
   a) A widespread group of Indians in southwest Texas and northern Mexico, whose history has been closely followed from 1582, perhaps as early as 1535, to about 1771. Before 1700 this group was allied with the Tejas Indians and the Spaniards, and at war with the Apaches. After 1700 they gradually became the allies of the Apaches and the enemies of their former friends, and were finally absorbed into the Apache group. They were closely related to the Patarabueyes of La Junta (by some accounts, identical) culturally, ethnically, and possibly linguistically. Eventually, those who were not absorbed into the Apaches were incorporated into the Conchos tribe. They may have been of Uto-Aztecan linguistic affiliation. In spite of the volume of evidence presented, some doubt has been expressed that any such specific Jumano group existed, in view of the facts noted below.
   b) The Quivira, or Wichita, Indians; or various subdivisions of this group later incorporated into the parent body; or to related peoples such as the Pawnee. All of these groups were *rayados* Indians. The name was also applied, in one isolated instance, to the Indians of a rancheria located in the vicinity of modern Flagstaff, Arizona, probably the Havasupai—apparently for the same reason as in the other cases, i.e., they were *rayados* (Bolton 1916:241).
   c) The outlying Tompiro pueblos of eastern New Mexico. These people were basically of Puebloan culture and were called Jumanos because of their trade relations with a group, or groups, of that name, and because some of their members were *rayados* Indians. Archaeological evidence in association with historical data indicates that these towns were an admixture of Puebloan culture with an older brown-ware

culture, presumably that of the Jumano group, partially incorporated into these settlements.

2) The name Jumano was apparently used by the Spaniards to mean *rayado*; hence, all *rayados* Indians were Jumanos. This would account for the various contradictory usages of the term and would answer many of the questions raised by earlier investigators. It would also throw doubt on the existence of any one Jumano tribe, from whom the name might originally have been derived.

The primary purpose of this study is to consider from both archaeological and historical viewpoints the Jumanos listed under item 1a above. Scholes's thesis regarding the use of "Jumano" in connection with tattooed Indians is completely convincing, and is accepted as an explanation of the designation of the eastern Pueblos, the Wichitas, and allied groups as Jumanos in the Spanish documentary sources. It will be shown, however, that there did exist a specific Indian group known to the Spaniards and the French, to other Indian groups, and probably among themselves as well, as Jumanos or some variation thereof. It will also be shown that these Jumanos are traceable as a group with characteristic culture, established geographical range, consistent relationships with other tribes (but subject to changes in political alignments), and under identical leadership in certain critical periods; and that the Jumanos, as such, were ethnically distinct from the Patarabueyes of La Junta, though culturally, politically, and possibly linguistically related to them. The respective cultures of the Jumanos and Patarabueyes will be summarized, their mutual relations at La Junta considered, and a brief analysis attempted of the peculiar and important function of the Jumanos in the development of aboriginal cultures in Texas and immediately adjoining areas.

Part II

Historical Data: The Jumanos

2

The Jumanos

1535(?)–1583

If the name Jumano was commonly applied in New Mexico to all *rayados* Indians, as Scholes has so convincingly demonstrated, the question arises as to the origin of the name. At present it is thought that it was first used by the historians of the Espejo expedition of 1582–1583. Luxán, whose day-by-day diary (translated in Hammond and Rey 1929) is the best available source regarding the expedition, applied the name to an Indian group encountered on the lower Pecos River, in the vicinity of Pecos, Texas. The rancherias of this group were scattered along a southern tributary of the Pecos, apparently Toyah Creek (Hammond and Rey 1929:124–25). They are here accepted as the original and true Jumanos, to whom the name should properly be applied and from whom it was presumably derived. By tracing the history and distribution of groups who were called Jumanos and who can be identified with this original group, the characteristics and identity of the true Jumanos will be ascertained.

In 1582 the Espejo expedition traveled down the Conchos River to La Junta and from there up the Rio Grande into New Mexico. Along the lower Conchos, at its junction with the Rio Grande, and for some distance above the junction, the Spaniards found sedentary villages of the Abriache and Otomoaco Indians, known collectively as the Patarabueyes. These Indians were *rayados* but in the Luxán diary they were not called Jumanos, although careful attention was given to the various La Junta tribes by name, and to their interrelationship (Luxán, in Hammond and Rey 1929:54–68; Espejo, in Bolton 1916:172–74). Espejo, however, in his account written from memory *after* the expedition's return to Mexico did not mention the various subdivisions noted by Luxán, but did state that

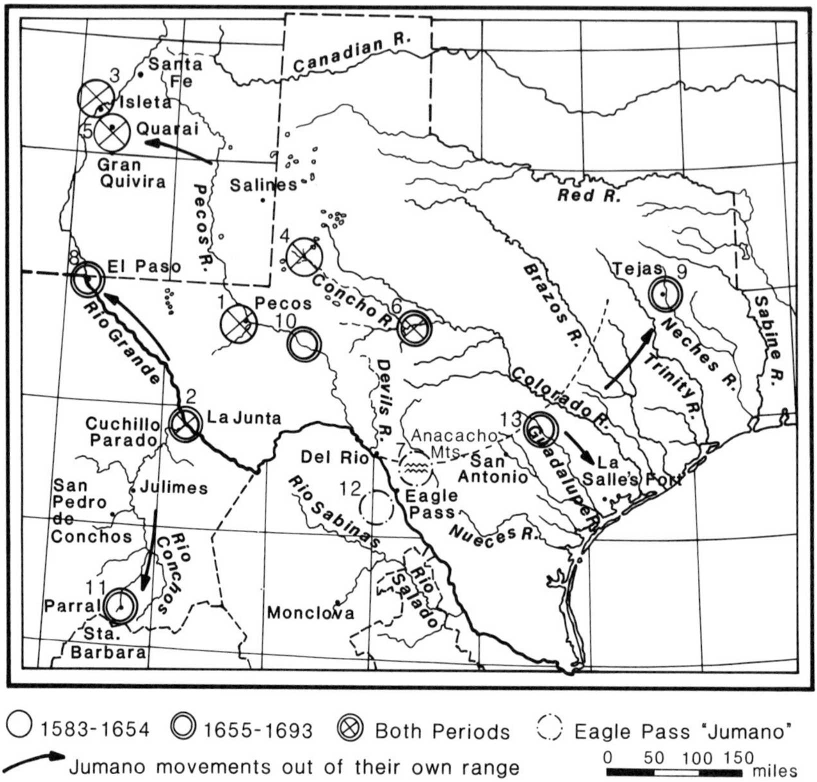

Figure 1. Known distribution of the Jumano Indians.

Patarabueye was another name for Jumano, the proper name for these Indians.[1] This seeming contradiction will be discussed at a later point.

The following year (1583) the Espejo expedition returned from New Mexico by way of the Pecos River (Rio de las Vacas). According to the Luxán diary, on August 7th the Spaniards encountered three "Jumanos" Indians (apparently the first recorded usage of the name) not far from modern Pecos, Texas. The Spaniards were able to understand the Jumanos through Pedro, a Patarabueye Indian traveling with Luxán. The Jumanos said that the Pecos, which they were following, flowed into the Rio Grande far below La Junta, but that they would guide the Spaniards to the Patarabueye Indians at La Junta by a good road. On the following day the Jumanos led the Spaniards to their rancheria on a small southwestern tributary of the Pecos, certainly Toyah Creek.[2] Here they were greeted with much music and rejoicing by many Jumano men and women, most of whom were en route to the large mesquite thickets on the Pecos River. A

Key to Figure 1.

1 Pecos and Toyah Creek
Jumanas. 1582. (Luxán, in Hammond and Rey 1929:124; Espejo, in Bolton 1916:189–90)

2 La Junta
Cumano Nation, Jumano. 1582(?)–1583. (Espejo, in Bolton 1916:172, 189–90)
Humana (or *Jumana*). 1683–1684. ("Declaration of Juan Sabeata," in "Viaje . . . ," Archivo General y Público, Mexico, Historia, Vol. 298)
Jumanes. 1684. (Posadas, in Duro 1882:56)

3 Isleta, New Mexico
Xumanas. 1629. (Vetancurt 1698:96–97; Hackett 1934:326)
Xumana. 1629. (Ayer 1916:57–58)

5 Quarai pueblo
Xumana. 1629. (Vetancurt 1698:189–90)

6 "Rio Nueces" (Concho River)
Xumanas. 1632. (Ayer 1916:58–62; Posadas, in Duro 1882:57)
Jumanas. 1650. (Posadas, in Duro 1882:57)
Jumanas. 1654. (Posadas, in Duro 1882:57–59)
Jumana. 1684. (Bolton 1916:320)

7 "Dacate" and "Sacatsol" mountains (identified by Bolton as Anacacho Mts.)
Xoman. 1675. (Bolton 1911:75)
Chomenes. 1688. (Bolton 1916:356–57)

8 El Paso
Jumana, Jumanes. 1683. ("Declaration of Juan Sabeata," in "Viaje . . . ," Archivo General y Público, Mexico, Historia, Vol. 298)

9 Tejas towns (Hasinai or Cenis villages)
Choumans. 1687. (Douay, in Cox 1915:234)

10 Rio Salado (Pecos)
Jumanas, Xumana, Jumanes. 1689. (Hackett 1926:256–62)

11 Parral, Chihuahua
Jumanas. 1689. (Hackett 1926:260)

12 South of the Rio del Norte (Rio Grande) in the general vicinity of Eagle Pass
Jumenes. 1689. (De León, in Bolton 1916:389)
Indians of the Frenchman. 1690. (De León, in Bolton 1916:406)
Chome. 1691. (Hatcher 1932:50)

13 Large spring on upper Guadalupe River, probably near New Braunfels, Texas
Chomanes, Chomas, Jumana, Jumanes. 1691. (Hatcher 1932:15)

---

dance was held by the Jumano men and women between their tents (*tiendas*). On succeeding days the Spaniards continued up Toyah Creek past San Solomon Springs at its head and into the Davis Mountains. All along this creek and at a rancheria in the mountains they found settled people of the Jumano nation. Luxán noted that the Jumanos were like the Patarabueyes in their style of clothing, but not in their houses.[3] The Jumano houses were skin tipis, while the houses of the Patarabueyes were large, rectangular jacale pithouses. In the Toyah Creek rancheria the Spaniards were given "delicious food," and in the rancheria in the mountains the Jumanos presented them with "raw and roasted calabashes and prickly pears." Led by their Jumano guides, the Spaniards continued through the mountains and plains of the Trans-Pecos region and finally reached the Rio Grande several leagues above a pueblo of the Patarabueye nation. The Jumanos were not again noted in the Luxán account.

The locations of the Jumanos described by the Espejo expedition historians are shown in Figure 1. The culture of this Jumano group, dismissing for the moment Espejo's designation of the Patarabueyes as Jumanos, may be summarized as follows:

Language. No data. Pedro, the Patarabueye interpreter was able to talk with them, but this is not necessarily evidence of linguistic relationship.

Economy. Hunting, and gathering of wild foods such as mesquite, calabashes (wild?), and prickly pear. Calabashes were served both raw and roasted.

Houses. "*Tiendas,*" probably pole and skin, or brush, tipis after the Plains style. Rancheria groupings along running streams and at springs.

Costume. Similar to that of the Patarabueyes.

Relations. Apparently friends and associates of the Patarabueyes.

General. They made music to greet the Spaniards and as a sign of peace both men and women performed a dance between the tents.

Previous investigators have identified as Jumanos an Indian tribe called the "People of the Cows" by Cabeza de Vaca. This was a sedentary agricultural group living in permanent houses along a river flowing between mountains. They went many leagues "up that river" to kill bison annually. Culturally, they sound very much like the Patarabueyes, with one exception, and their country was similar to that of La Junta (de Vaca, in Bandelier 1905:149–55, and in Hodge 1907:3–126). These factors, along with the fact that the Patarabueyes (or the Jumanos visiting there) told the Espejo party that Cabeza de Vaca had been among them (Luxán, in Hammond and Rey 1929:62), are responsible for the initial identification of the People of the Cows as Patarabueyes, and, after the Espejo expedition, as Jumanos.

Hallenbeck (1940:194–215), however, has raised serious objections to routing de Vaca through La Junta, and an even more serious objection has arisen from the archaeological evidence. Cabeza de Vaca noted that the People of the Cows boiled their food in gourd vessels by placing hot rocks in the stew therein, since they had no pots in which to cook in the ordinary manner.[4] As a result of the intensive archaeological work at La Junta, it is known that the occupants of the La Junta villages apparently had pottery from about the thirteenth century until they were absorbed by the Spaniards. This seems to eliminate de Vaca's description of the People of the Cows as an early reference to the Patarabueyes, whether the latter were Jumanos or not.

One solution is that the People of the Cows may actually have been

Jumanos, though not Patarabueyes. We have no historical reference to pottery among the Jumanos, and the river flowing between mountains may have been the Pecos, up which they went for more than forty leagues to kill the cattle; or it may have been the Rio Grande near El Paso, as Hallenbeck (1940:210) thinks. Hallenbeck also notes that Indians in northwestern Texas (probably along the rimrock of the high plains or in Palo Duro canyon) when visited by Coronado's army in 1541 piled their goods in a heap, as the Indians previously visited by de Vaca had done. Coronado's men did not ignore the goods as de Vaca had done, however, and the Indians were angered. As he notes, this custom was observed only among the Indians along the Rio Grande. Another Indian informed the Spaniards that others like them had been seen, but further to the west. Since the upper headwaters of the Concho and the Colorado rivers in Texas were Jumano territory, as will be shown, the Jumanos may not only have been the ones visited by de Vaca, but also those encountered by Coronado's group and those who told the Espejo party of having seen de Vaca. This is an interesting and ingenious explanation of otherwise contradictory data, but it is unfortunately not subject to proof.

3

The Jumanos

1584–1654

After the Espejo *entrada* no reference to the Jumanos can be found until about 1623. The Jumano pueblos of the Salinas region were visited by Oñate in 1598,[1] but as Scholes has shown, these were Tompiro-speaking Pueblo towns, called Jumano because of the application of this name to all *rayados* Indians and because "Jumanos" from the plains came there to trade (Scholes and Mera 1940). The Oñate expedition also noted the application of the name Jumano to a Wichita group by the Christian Indians of New Mexico, in the sense of their being *rayados.*[2] Also in 1598, Captain Farfán de los Godos (in Bolton 1916:241), sent by Oñate to the west and southwest of the Hopi towns in northeastern Arizona, applied the name "Jumana" to a group of Indians found there. All these instances are obviously connected with the usage of the term for people with body decoration, and none of them seem to refer to the true Jumanos.

Some six years before 1629, Fray Juan de Salas traveled among the Tompiros in the Salinas region and encountered the Jumano Indians. The Jumanos were so impressed with his conduct that they begged him to stay with them (Ayer 1916:58). They continued to beg for missionaries and finally in July of 1629 a delegation of fifty Jumanos visited Isleta, New Mexico, and told the priests of a beautiful woman who had appeared to them and instructed them to make this visit, and again they requested that priests be sent among them (Vetancurt 1698:96–97; see also translation in Hackett 1934:326). Impressed by this vision, Fray Salas and Fray Diego Lopez accompanied the Jumanos for some 112 leagues to the east (in the Vetancurt account, over 100 leagues to the *north,* which is obviously a mistake) where they found the main Jumano tribe celebrating "one of their customary feasts." The Jumanos received the priests well, and many of them claimed to have been miraculously cured during their visit. They asked for baptism and placed crosses over the doors of their homes. Since the Jumanos were at war with the Apaches, their location was not a permanent one; therefore, the priests induced the Indians to accompany them to a place near Quarai pueblo in New Mexico, where the priests administered to them (Vetancurt 1698).

According to Benavides (Ayer 1916:57–58), at this time the territory of the Jumanos lay 112 leagues to the east of Santa Fe, between the territory of the Vaquero Apaches and the great salt lakes of eastern New Mexico, or more probably on the south Panhandle salt lakes, where the Salineros Indians lived on the Pecos River. This general location would seem actually to have been southeast rather than east, since a location of 112 leagues to the east would not border on the Salines region and the Salineros Indians. This was a temporary Jumano camp, as indicated by Benavides, probably located in the north Concho or Colorado River drainage, on the plains east of Carlsbad, and not far from the spot where they were originally found by the Espejo expedition. These Jumanos were also neighbors of the Iapes and the Xabateas, and some thirty leagues to the east of them were found the Quiviras and the Aixaos (Aijados-Taovayas?). These Jumanos were perpetually at war with the Vaquero Apaches, and presumably were the Jumanos whose frequent trading expeditions to Gran Quivira helped secure for it the name of the "Pueblo of the Jumanos" (Ayer 1916; Scholes and Mera 1940:280).

Apparently the Jumanos did not long remain peacefully settled at Quarai, for in 1632 Fray Salas and Fray Diego de Ortega, with some soldiers, visited them again. This time they were found 200 leagues southeast of Santa Fe and some 80 leagues east of La Junta on a river ("Rio Nueces") luxuriant with mulberry trees, plums, wild grapes, many nut trees (perhaps pecan), and where there were many buffalo, deer, and wild turkeys (Posadas, in Duro 1882:57). Bolton identified this river as the present Concho River near San Angelo, Texas; Pichardo had earlier placed the river in the same general location (Bolton 1911:69–71; see also Pichardo's map in Hackett 1934). The priests and soldiers were received in friendship by the Jumanos, who again showed an inclination to become Christians. Salas returned to Santa Fe, but Ortega remained there for six months among the Jumanos and was not harmed. Apparently the Jumano rancheria on the "Rio Nueces" was more than just a temporary camp. (The "Rio Nueces" of historical accounts may be, as Bolton thought, the modern-day Concho River in Texas, an upper branch of the Colorado, but this has never been proven. In fact, the archaeological evidence, or lack of it, on the Concho suggests that other explanations for the location of the historical "Rio Nueces" should at least be considered.* For that reason, the name "Rio Nueces" has been preserved throughout this study; it is not to be confused with the modern Nueces River.)

We next hear of this particular Jumano group in 1560. At that time an expedition under Captain Hernan Martin and Captain Diego del Castillo went 200 leagues to the same Rio Nueces, but by a different route, and remained among the Jumanos there for some six months, owing to an abundance of provisions and because of the discovery of pearls in the river. Following downstream to the east along the Rio Nueces, the Spaniards passed through the land of the Cuitoas (Kichai?), the Escanjaques (Yscanis?), and the Aijados (identified by Hodge as the Taovayas, a Wichita subgroup), and after 50 leagues came to the border of the country of the Tejas Indians (Posados, in Duro 1882:57).

This expedition returned to Santa Fe, where the pearls found in the Rio Nueces caused much excitement. The pearls were sent to Mexico and, as a result, an order was dispatched to Santa Fe ordering another expedition to explore and map the Rio Nueces and surrounding country and record all pertinent facts about it. As a result, in 1654 a new expeditionary force of thirty soldiers and two hundred Christian Indians, under the leadership of Don Diego de Guadalajara, visited the Rio Nueces at a point some 200 leagues from Santa Fe. On arriving there, they were told by the Jumanos that the Cuitoas, Escanjaques, and Aijados were at war. Accompanied by the Jumanos and the Christian Indians, Guadalajara marched 30 leagues to the east, where he fought a battle with the Cuitoas and defeated them before the Escanjaques, who were rushing to their aid, could arrive. Armed with spoils in the form of many bundles of deer and buffalo skins and two hundred prisoners, the party returned to the post of the Jumanos on the Rio Nueces, where the Spanish soldiers had remained. The party then returned to Santa Fe. It was noted, significantly as we shall see, that a soldier named Juan Dominguez de Mendoza was a member of the expedition (Posadas, in Duro 1882:57).

Thus, from 1632 to 1654, Indians known as Jumanos were found on the "Rio Nueces" of west-central Texas, where they had a more or less permanent focus of settlement; the Spaniards continually found them there, and on two occasions the Spaniards remained for a period of six months with them in this location. Earlier, possibly as early as 1623, they were found in the same general region. The Jumanos of 1632, 1650, and 1654 were obviously the same group, since they were found in the same location, under the same name, apparently had the same general cultural characteristics, the same political relations, and reacted to the Spaniards in the same way in each instance. The Jumanos of 1632 were probably

*Recent field work on the Concho has proved almost conclusively that the "Rio Nueces" of Spanish documents is the Concho River. See p. 108. (J.C.K.)

identical to the earlier group visited by Salas in 1629 and earlier, for the same reasons, and were obviously so considered by Salas. Although the Toyah Creek Jumanos of the Espejo expedition were found farther to the south and west than the Jumanos of the 1623–1654 period, the cultural characteristics noted appear to have been identical, and the name is the same. In the next section, definite evidence of the identification of the groups of the two periods will be presented.

The cultural traits of the Jumanos of the period of 1623–1654 may be summarized as follows:

Language. No data.

Economy. Principally buffalo hunters, following the herds wherever they roamed, although they possessed fairly permanent settlements on the Rio Nueces. It is inferred that they were also gatherers of wild plants, such as plums, mulberries, grapes, and nuts. Portable tipis ("and so the captains ordered that they should strike their tents to go the next day at dawn"); above the doors of the front of the tents the Indians placed crosses after receiving religious instruction (Ayer 1916:58–62).

Costume. No data.

Relations. Continuously at war with the Vaquero Apaches, and at times with the Cuitoas, Escanjaques, and Aijados. Friends and neighbors of the Iapes, Xabateas, and possibly of the Salineros, Quiviras, and Tejas. They traded (presumably) with the Tompiros of Gran Quivira, and were friendly with the Spaniards.

Range. Centered about the "Rio Nueces" in west-central Texas, but roamed over the plains south and east of the Vaquero Apaches, following the buffalo. They visited Gran Quivira and Isleta pueblos in New Mexico, and apparently were found at one time in the Carlsbad region. Their territory was bounded on the northwest by the Salinas country of southeastern New Mexico, and by the Salineros Indians of the Pecos River; on the north by the Vaquero Apaches; on the east and southeast by the Quiviras, Aijados, Cuitoas, Escanjaques, and Tejas. They were also neighbors of the Iapes, Xabateas, and others whose location is not given. Their boundary and range on the south and west is not stated.

General. They were very friendly with the Spaniards and desired to become Christians. They adopted the sign of the cross and were adept at telling the Spaniards of miraculous visions and visitations to enlist their interest. From 1623 on, they were subject to religious training by the Spanish priests. Benavides speaks of "Indian sorcerers" (Ayer 1916:59). There is a strong implication that they were *rayados,* or tattooed Indians, although no definite statement to this effect is made.

4
The Jumanos
1655–1693

Presumably the Spaniards remained in constant touch with the Jumanos on the Rio Nueces (probably the present Concho River; see pages 20 and 108 after 1654, since the authorities wrote in 1683, referring to the Jumanos of the Rio Nueces: "before 1680, when the Pueblo revolt had occurred, trade and friendship had been maintained with the Jumanos 'with such security that the Spaniards, six, eight, and ten, went to their lands and villages every year to trade with these Indians' in buckskins, *teccas*[?], and buffalo hides" (Bolton 1912:11). No recorded expedition visited them again, however, until 1683.

In 1683 several Indian delegations appeared at El Paso del Norte requesting missionaries. The last of these delegations arrived in October. It consisted of a Jumano Indian named Juan Sabeata and six followers. Sabeata asked for missionaries, stating that 33 tribes, including the Jumanos, desired baptism. To give weight to his request, he told the priests at El Paso of the miraculous appearance of a cross, to which they had supplicated when hard-pressed in battle. This cross was placed on their standard, and the battle was won without the loss of a single life, and much booty was gained. Realizing that this was a miracle, they had come at once seeking baptism. Much later the Spaniards learned that this story had been made up by a Tejas Indian in order that the Spaniards might help him return from La Junta to his home in east Texas across the territory of the warring Apaches (Posadas, in Duro 1882:56).

Sabeata said that he himself lived at La Junta with many of his own people and Julimes Indians. Part of his tribe, "the extended nation of the Humanas," lived six days' travel eastward from La Junta; three days' travel eastward were the buffalo herds and three days beyond was the Rio Nueces, the home of some of the Jumanos and many other friendly tribes. From La Junta to the Tejas Indians it was fifteen or twenty days' travel. Two Tejas Indian messengers awaited him at La Junta at that time (Hackett 1931:137–41).

Fray Nicolás Lopez previously had heard at Parral that Indians from La Junta came there asking for missionaries, which, however, had been denied them, owing to the great distance between Parral and La Junta. He was, therefore, favorably impressed with their request, but to test their ardor he told them that a church would be needed. The Indians sent messengers to measure the El Paso church and altar, and returned speedily to La Junta to see that churches were built. In twenty days sixty Indian men and women, some of whom had worked at Parral, returned saying that two churches were being built (Hackett 1934:349–52).

Impressed with the serious attitude of the Indians, Fray Lopez and two other priests accompanied them back to La Junta, going on foot for thirteen days and passing through the land of the Suma Indians. Arriving at the first of the La Junta nations, the priests found a large church of grass, with an altar the dimensions of that at El Paso, already constructed (Hackett 1934:349–52). Six leagues farther on, apparently at La Junta itself, they found a second church, larger and better built, and a house built for the residence of the priests. It was discovered that many of the La Junta Indians had already become Christians (Duro 1882:68).

Seven other of the La Junta nations later built churches (four, according to another source). In all, nine nations were found at La Junta, among others the Julimes, Jumanos, Rayados, Oposmes, Polumes, Polulanas, and Polaques. Many other neighboring nations came to request religious attention. The La Junta tribes were settled and some of them sowed quantities of corn, wheat, beans, calabashes, watermelons, cantaloupes, and tobacco. Over five hundred Indians were baptized at La Junta at this time (Hackett 1934:349–52, 1937:360–63; Posadas, in Duro 1882:56).

In December, Juan Dominguez de Mendoza came down the Rio Grande from El Paso with a group of soldiers. He had been instructed to attempt "the new discovery of the Jumanas and all other nations who hold friendship with them," and the "Discovery of the East and the Kingdom of the Texas" (see "Itinerary of... Mendoza," in Bolton 1916:320–43). This was the same Juan Dominguez de Mendoza who had accompanied the Guadalajara expedition of 1654 to the Rio Nueces and the Jumanos. At La Junta the expedition was joined by Fray Lopez and one of the other priests, Fray Juan Zavaleta, leaving the other priest, Fray Antonio Acevedo, to administer to the new La Junta missions (Bolton 1916:316).

The party was led by Juan Sabeata and his Jumanos but included Indians of other nations as well. Traveling northward, the expedition reached the Pecos River ("Rio Salado") after 70 leagues of travel. After going down the Pecos for nine leagues, the party traveled eastward 40 leagues to the headwaters of the Rio de Señor San Pedro (Middle Concho), and down it, still eastward, 24 leagues to the junction with the "Rio Nueces," or "Rio Perlas." Mendoza noted that this spot was about eight leagues farther down the Rio Nueces than the place where he had been with the Guadalajara expedition in 1654. The party continued eastward down the Rio Nueces until they reached a large river, the "San Clemente," obviously the Colorado River where they remained for six weeks awaiting a large number of other tribes and subject to continual attacks by the Apaches. Here they killed over four thousand buffalo. Finally the Apache attacks grew so strong that the Spaniards sent word to the Indians that they would come again at a later date, and returned to La Junta. There Fray Acevedo stayed to help administer the La Junta missions, and Mendoza and Lopez returned to El Paso by way of the Rio Conchos (of Chihuahua) and the Rio Sacramento, bypassing the Sumas along the Rio Grande who had revolted in their absence. Juan Sabeata and his Jumanos fell into disfavor with the Spaniards and with the assembled Indians, and did not accompany the party back to La Junta (Bolton 1916:336–39).

As Bolton has pointed out, the Mendoza expedition is the key to the entire Jumano problem. In the first place, it enables an identification of the seventeenth century Rio Nueces as a branch of the Concho River, since Mendoza's diary enables a clear tracing of his route from La Junta eastward (see Smith 1928 for a discussion of the Mendoza route). Furthermore, Mendoza, who was a member of the earlier expedition, specifically states that this was the same Rio Nueces as that reached in the 1654 *entrada,* and consequently by the earlier *entradas* as well.

Not only does the Mendoza expedition identify the Rio Nueces, it also identifies the Jumanos of 1632–1654 as the Jumanos of 1683–1684, and the Jumanos of the Rio Nueces as those of La Junta and the intervening regions, including, without doubt, the Toyah Creek Jumanos of 1583. We have Sabeata's own statement, in addition to the facts of the expedition, as to the identity of the eastern and western Jumano groups. We also have Sabeata's own reference to his people as "the extended nation of the Humanas," indicating that the name was at least known and accepted by the Jumanos as their own group name, whether or not it originated with them. This is further indicated by the accounts of the La Salle expedition in Texas, discussed later. Supporting the concept of a specific Jumano group is the statement made by Fray Lopez after his return to El Paso, to the effect that he had learned the Jumano language, had developed a very large vocabulary in it, and had preached to the Jumanos in their own language. One of the other priests had also learned the Jumano language:

> For he has already communicated with and knows the said nations, and is acquainted with the Jumana language and has preached in it to those barbarians, having a very large vocabulary in the said tongue, as has been legally declared [by those who] have heard him preach; and one of the religious he took as companion was already skilled in it, though not in full perfection. [Hackett 1937:362]

Jumano relationships at La Junta are also clarified. Although the Jumanos are mentioned as a La Junta group, and Sabeata stated that some of his people lived there, at least eight other groups are mentioned also as native tribes of La Junta, and Mendoza states specifically that the farming settlements at La Junta itself were those of the Julimes Indians (Bolton 1916:325). Furthermore, the Jumanos did not accompany the Spaniards back to La Junta, although the settlements there had remained intact, a priest had continued the religious activities of the missions, and on stopping at La Junta on the return trip Mendoza gave "rods of justice" (canes of authority) to four of the chiefs there (Bolton 1916:317).

Perhaps one of the most important conclusions derived from the accounts of the Mendoza expedition is the identification of the Jumanos of the Rio Nueces, the La Junta region, and intervening areas, as those under the leadership of Juan Sabeata. Although the conclusion of the expedition found Sabeata in disfavor with both Spaniards and Indians, according to Mendoza, he nevertheless remained leader of the Jumanos and certain allied tribes; from 1683 to 1692 we are able to trace the widespread movements of the tribe, and make certain identification of groups called Jumanos because of his appearance in the Spanish accounts as their leader. Sabeata was, in fact, one of the most widely known Indians of Texas in the seventeenth century.

Although Sabeata had stated that some of his people lived on the Rio Nueces, the only Jumanos noted there by the Mendoza expedition in 1684 were those under Sabeata who had accompanied the party from La Junta. It seems probable that the Rio Nueces settlements were being deserted by the Jumanos at this time, owing to increasing pressure from the Apaches to the north. This was clearly stated by Fray Alonzo Posadas in 1686. After describing the series of expeditions to the Jumanos on the Rio Nueces from 1632 to 1684, Posadas defined the range of the various tribes, locating the Apaches on the plains north of the Rio Nueces, and noting that the Jumanos and other tribes had been dispossessed of the Rio Nueces and driven back to their present location on the Rio del Norte (Duro 1882:62).

Probably responsible for the Jumano petition for missionaries in 1683 and the resulting Mendoza expedition was the Jumanos' hope that the Spaniards could be induced to drive the Apaches back from the Rio Nueces. Shortly after the Mendoza party had reached the Pecos River, Sabeata, acting as representative of the Jumanos and associated tribes, asked Mendoza to make war on the Apaches. This request was granted, to the joy of the Indians. On several occasions the Jumanos reported to Mendoza that the Apaches were near and induced him to stop and fight them. Mendoza became angered with the continual efforts of Sabeata to embroil him in battles with the Apaches, accusing him of falsehood in the matter. While in the vicinity of the Rio Nueces, the Mendoza party was actually attacked on several occasions by the Apaches demonstrating their strength in that region (Bolton 1916:331–38).

In 1687, while among the Teao, apparently on the lower Colorado River, La Salle's party heard of the Choumenes (or "Chaumenes") as one of the tribes through whose territory they had passed en route from the French fort on the Garcetas River, just off Matagorda Bay.[1] The Teao themselves had been among the Spaniards. A day's journey farther northeast the French stopped at the rancheria of the Palaquechaune ("Palaquesson" in Douay's account) Indians. These Indians told the French that they were "allies to the Cenis [Hasinai, Tejas], that their chief had been among the Choumans, who were Friends to the Spaniards, from whom they got Horses" and that "the Choumans had given their Chief some presents to persuade him to conduct the French to them; that most of the said Nation had flat Heads; that they had Indian Corn. . . ."[2]

Among the Cenis, the French found many items that had been obtained from the Spaniards: dollars, silver spoons, lace, clothes, horses, and even "a bull from Rome exempting the Spaniards in Mexico from fasting during summer" (Douay, in Cox 1905:232–33). Douay noted that the Tejas

> have intercourse with the Spaniards through the Choumans, their allies, who are always at war with New Spain. . . . They reckoned themselves six days' journey from the Spaniards, of whom they gave us so natural a description that we no longer had any doubts on the point, although the Spaniards had not yet undertaken to come to their villages, their warriors merely joining the Choumans to go war on New Mexico. [Douay, in Cox 1905:233]

The Jumanos and Cibolas themselves later told the Spaniards that the Tejas Indians were eight or more days' travel from La Junta, the easternmost Spanish outpost. Regarding the statement that the Choumans were at war with the Spaniards (New Spain and New Mexico), it will be recalled that the Mendoza expedition parted from the Jumanos in 1684 in great anger, accusing the Indians of having plotted to kill them. Also, shortly after the return of the expedition, open rebellion flared in the Patarabueye towns at La Junta, and the Spaniards were forced to leave, abandoning the missions. The state of warfare was a temporary one, however, as implied in Douay's own account of the close trade relations between the Choumans and Spaniards. Douay continues:

> There were then some Chouman ambassadors among them, who came to visit us. I was agreeably surprised to see them make the sign of the cross, kneel, clasp their hands, and raise them from time to time to heaven. They also kissed my habit, and gave me to understand that men dressed like us instructed tribes in their vicinity, who were only two days' march from the Spaniards, where our religious had large churches, in which all assembled to pray. They expressed very naturally the ceremonies of the mass; one of them sketched me a painting that he had seen of a great lady, who was weeping because her son was upon a cross. He told us that the Spaniards butchered the Indians cruelly, and, finally, that if we would go with them, or give them guns, they could easily conquer them, because they were a cowardly race, who had no courage, and made people walk before them with a fan to refresh them in hot weather. [Douay, in Cox 1905:234–35]

De Lisle listed the "Choumay" among the friends and allies of the Cadodaquious (Caddos) lying to the southwest of the Caddo towns on the Red River (Joutel, in Margry 1878:408–10) and in 1691 Fray Francisco Casanas de Jesús María listed the "Chuman" as one of the allies of the Hasinai lying some 80 leagues to the south and west (Hatcher 1926:206–18). The Spanish spelling of Jumano varies considerably, ranging through Choma, Xoman, Juman, and Jumane, and there is convincing evidence that the Choumane, Chumay, and Chuman, listed as friends and allies of the Tejas (Hasinai), were identical to the Jumanos of La Junta and the Rio Nueces.

In 1688 the Spaniards at Parral received word from La Junta de los Rios that some Cibola and Jumano Indians had reported that "strange Spaniards" (actually the French under La Salle) were traveling among the Indians of Texas. As a result, a series of investigations was held, and an expedition journeyed as far as the Pecos River to investigate the reports. The testimony of the various Spaniards and Indians involved throws much light on the activities of the Jumano Indians and on their relations with the Indians of La Junta. The accounts are long and repetitious, but owing to the importance of the data included they are presented here, in the form of excerpts and summaries, in some detail. The source of the accounts summarized below is Hackett (1926:234–61). In the original testimonies, the Indians refer to the French as "Spaniards," or occasionally "Moors." In the paraphrase below, "French" has been substituted, since that is clearly who the "strange Spaniards" were.

At the beginning of the investigations in November, 1688, Don Nicolás, governor of the Julimes Indians, traveled with his people from La Junta to San Francisco de Conchos where the first inquiries were held. Don Nicolás stated that there were some friendly Cibola Indians at the Rio del Norte and that the Julimes of La Junta traded and bargained with them. These Cibolas were messengers sent by the Cibola chief[3] to inform the La Junta Indians that he was coming there with his people, and that he was bringing with him a Frenchman who had become separated from those who were marching near the Tejas Indians (La Salle's party). The messengers also said that the Cibola chief was bringing letters from the French. Don Nicolás states further that on other occasions he had heard the Cibolas and their captain say that the French were going among the Tejas and giving them axes in exchange for horses (Hackett 1926:234–36).

Juan de Salaises, an Indian who accompanied Don Nicolás, corroborated his chief's testimony, stating in more detail that the French were "travelling in the neighborhood of the Cibolos Indians, who come from the direction of the east to trade and bargain with them [the Julimes of La Junta] as friends, as they are . . . " (Hackett 1926:237–39).

In the same month, Fray Agustín de Colina, president of the missions of La Junta, and Fray Joachim de Hinojosa, one of the La Junta missionaries, testified at the pueblo of San Pedro de Conchos regarding their knowledge of the reported French *entrada*. Fray Colina declared that in 1687 the Jumano and Cibola Indians asked him for a letter to give to the French who were traveling among the Tejas. He told them to bring a letter to him from the strangers and he would answer it. In September of 1688, five Cibola Indians came to La Junta and visited him at the mission. They told him of the French who had joined them. Afterwards, other Cibola Indians arrived and told in some detail of the strangers dressed in armor, who slept nights on their ships, one of which had been sunk, and who traded with the Tejas and other tribes (Hackett 1926:241–43).

Alarmed by these accounts, the authorities dispatched Captain Juan Fernandez de Retana to La Junta with orders to investigate the stories further, and if possible to cross the Rio del Norte and reconnoiter the French camp. Along the way, he was to make war upon several of the rebellious tribes between Parral and La Junta (Hackett 1926:241–43). When Retana arrived at La Junta in 1689 he sent out "the most experienced Indians of the country" to explore the region beyond the Rio del Norte through which he would have to travel. A few days later, the scouts returned, bringing "news that they had heard that a governor to whom these nations [the Jumanos and Cibolas] are subject was already en route from the Texas Indians and that he would give . . . an account of everything." After some delay, Retana grew impatient and went out to meet the Indians. Four days' journey beyond the Rio del Norte from La Junta, apparently on the Rio Salado (Pecos River), he "met the said governor, whose name is Don Juan Xaviata, and who is the principal chief of the Cibolo and Jumano nations." Sabeata reported that the French settlement had been destroyed by the Indians of the region, but that a few of the Frenchmen still survived and were hiding among the Tejas Indians. Sabeata himself carried some papers in French and a necklace of wide lace which had been obtained from the Indians who had destroyed the settlement. According to Sabeata, it was an eighteen-day wagon journey from the Rio Salado to the Tejas (Hackett 1926:257–59).

On receiving this information from Retana, the authorities ordered that Sabeata be brought to Parral for examination, and "since there is no interpreter of the Cibolo and Jumano languages in this camp, he shall order Don Nicolás, governor of the Julimes nation, and one other who also understands them, to come with [Don Juan Sabeata]" (Hackett 1926: 259–61).

In April, 1689, Sabeata's party arrived at Parral. It consisted of Sabeata himself, "who said that he was governor of the Indians of the Cibolos and Jumanos nations, and Miguel, who said that he was captain of the said nations that reside on the Rio del Norte, and other caciques [Cuis Benive and Muygisofac, both Cibolas], who said that they are heathens and that they live at their rancherias on the lower Rio del Norte" (Hackett 1926:261).[4] Don Nicolás, the Julimes, served as interpreter.

These Indians stated that they had heard good reports of the Spaniards at Parral from some of the La Junta Indians and "that they would have come earlier but for the fact that the time for going into the interior to the fairs[5] which they conduct with the nations of the upper Rio del Norte,[6] the Texas, and many other Indian nations, prevented them from doing so." They affirmed that the French had been destroyed, and turned over to the Spaniards two sheets of paper from a French book, a parchment with a painting of a ship and written annotations in French, and a neckcloth of lace (Hackett 1926:261).[7]

The Julimes Indians under Don Nicolás lived at La Junta,[8] and some of them went at times to work in the Spanish plantations farther up the Rio Conchos.[9] Friendly Jumano and Cibola Indians came from the east to trade with the Julimes and to receive religious instruction at the La Junta missions.[10] Don Nicolás, the Julimes chief, was able to speak the language of the Cibolas and Jumanos (it will be remembered that he served as an interpreter for them in dealings with the Spaniards) some of whom lived the year around at La Junta.[11] Others of the Cibolas (and Jumanos?) apparently spent the entire year in rancherias along the Colorado River from the Rio Nueces (Concho) almost to the coast, and probably along the nearby Guadalupe River and similar streams. Still other Jumanos and Cibolas, probably the main group of these Indians, were seasonal nomads, spending the winter in the La Junta settlements, but leaving in the early spring to go to the hunting grounds in central Texas, where they remained until the fall of the year, at which time they returned to La Junta.

Although the Jumanos and Cibolas were under the leadership of Juan Sabeata, they had other minor captains, such as Miguel, the Cibola (Hackett 1926:269–73).[12] En route to the hunting grounds in the spring they went from La Junta through the mountains (Davis Mountains?) to the Pecos River and on to the Rio Nueces.[13] From there the country was open and they visited various places in central, east, and south Texas, including the rancherias of the Tejas Indians, those of the "Sierra" (probably the rancherias along the Balcones Escarpment), and those near the sea coast.[14] Although the trip from La Junta to the Tejas was spoken of, perhaps boastfully, as a short one, estimated at eight to twelve days of sunrise to sunset travel, they normally took much more time in making it, going with caution and making side trips to the rancherias of many Indian nations to talk and gather news.[15] This is an important sidelight on the dynamics of diffusion of news, and hence potentially of other cultural items as well, among the aboriginal Texans. Annual fairs were held among the Tejas Indians, the Indians of the various Texas rivers, and many other Indian nations. The Jumanos regularly attended these fairs.[16]

At certain times of the year, buffalo wandered into the plains between the Rio Nueces and the Rio del Norte until the country was filled with them. Every year the Jumanos and Cibolas had wars with certain "Caribe" Indians, probably Apaches, over the killing of these animals, which migrated from place to place to find new pasture (Hackett 1926:273–77).

The Cibola villages on the lower Colorado River were visited by the French on several occasions, and the French questioned them about the Spanish. The Jumanos and Cibolas also were visiting in the Tejas towns at least twice when the French were there, and talked to them at those times; on the last occasion one of the surviving French started out with them to La Junta but changed his mind and returned.[17] These various meetings between the French and the Cibolas and Jumanos on the lower Colorado River and in the Tejas towns suggest those described in the accounts of Joutel and Douay. This is one point indicating the identity of Jumanos and Choumans.

The exact meetings described in the testimonies are apparently not the same, however. Thus, the Cibolas and Jumanos at Parral noted that when the French visited their village in central Texas they came up the river in canoes, whereas in the meetings described by Joutel and Douay, the French traveled across country and forded the rivers or crossed them on crude homemade boats and rafts. Nevertheless, it is highly important that the French tell of meeting the friends and allies of the "Choumans" who had intercourse with the Spaniards, while the Jumanos later tell the Spaniards of meetings between their friends and allies, the Cibolas, and the French in central Texas, in both instances apparently on the lower Colorado River. Perhaps significantly, the allies of the Choumans on the lower Colorado were identified as the Palaquesson; one of the important La Junta groups was the Polaques, sometimes known as "Sibolas de Polaques," and it was the Cibolas who were visited by the French.

Similarly, the meetings betweeen Jumanos and French described by Douay are not the identical ones noted by the Jumanos and Cibolas at Parral, since the latter occurred after the destruction of the French fort and the former was prior to its destruction. Again there is the impressive fact, however, that both sides report meetings with the other.

In June, 1691, the Teran-Massanet expedition stopped at a rancheria of the Payaya Indians in south-central Texas, probably near San Antonio. The Payaya offered to guide the Spaniards to the rancherias of the Choma[18] Indians. After traveling toward the northeast for some 18 to 21 leagues, the party arrived at the Choma rancherias located in a wood near one of the springs that form the Guadalupe River, probably a few miles up the river from modern New Braunfels, Texas. A few miles from the rancheria they were met by a welcoming delegation consisting of the captains of the Chomas, the Cibolas, the Chalomes, the Cantonas, the Guanayas (Canayas, Chaynayas), and the Catquezas and their peoples. Teran included the "Mandones" in this group.[19] The captain of the Chomas was "Don Juan Sabiata." The entire group was estimated to number about two thousand Indians. All those who came to meet the Spaniards were on horseback, "mounted on very small saddles which resembled riding saddles with stirrups. When asked where they got these little saddles, they [said] they had taken them from the Apaches in war." The captains carried crosses of wood before them and the captains of the Cibolas and the Catquezas carried an image of "Our Lady of Guadalupe." The captain of the Catqueza tribe, Nicolás, was "well versed in the Mexican dialects and in the Spanish language."[20] He had been reared in Parral (Saltillo and Parral) but had returned to live with his own people, where he enjoyed the respect of all the surrounding tribes because of his ability. Don Sabeata and his lieutenants carried commissions issued in Nueva Vizcaya.

The Indians gave the Spaniards letters written by the Spanish missionaries among the Tejas and entrusted to them for delivery. After talking with the captains, Massanet wrote:

> The above mentioned nations, the Choma, Cibola and Canaya are Indians who live in and about the country along the banks of the Rio del Norte. They border on the Salineros Indians who live on the banks of the Salado, a river that runs into the Rio del Norte. They also border upon the Apaches with whom they are often at war. The Apaches live in a mountain range which runs from east to west. They are at war with all the other nations, except the Salineros with whom they are at peace . . . In the end they dominate all the other Indians. The Chomas are the same Indians who in Parral and New Mexico are called Jumanes. Every year they come to the headwaters of the Guadalupe River and sometimes as far as the Tejas country. They come to kill buffaloes and carry away the skins, because in their country there are no buffaloes. When it gets cold they return to their own country. [Massanet, in Hatcher 1932:58–59]

The "mountain range which runs from east to west" in which the Apaches lived was probably the Cap Rock of the High Plains, although its general trend is north and south, or possibly the Balcones Escarpment, but this seems too far south for the Apache range at this period.

Massanet talked for some time with Sabeata and Nicolás, both of whom tried to induce him to remain among their people, many of whom they said were Christians, having been baptized in Parral and El Paso. Massanet put them off, however, remarking that "if they really wanted missionaries in their country, they doubtless would have had them before this, as they go to Parral and Paso de Nuevo Mexico every year" (Hatcher 1932:58–59).

Juan Sabeata and his people followed the expedition for some days recovering and returning to the Spaniards, in one instance, a herd of lost horses, but the Spaniards nevertheless grew suspicious of them. Other Indians, of the Pacpule and Quema nations warned the party that the Jumanos intended to murder them, so after keeping close watch all night, the Spaniards sent the Jumanos away on the following day, after presenting Sabeata with a rifle and ammunition (Hatcher 1932:63–64). So, as he had previously with the Mendoza expedition, Sabeata gained the suspicions and mistrust of the party.

This verifies the identification of the Choumans of eastern and southern Texas with the Jumanos of west Texas, and supplements the information on the movements of the Jumanos and on their alliances gleaned from the Parral testimonies.

In July of the following year, 1692, Juan Sabeata again appeared in Parral, bringing with him a letter from the Spanish missionaries among the Tejas. The letter had been written on September 4, 1690, and was addressed to the missionaries at El Paso. Sabeata was required to testify again in regard to his travels and the distances between La Junta and the Tejas. He stated that he went to the Tejas to investigate reports of strangers there, but finding only the Spanish priests who gave him the letter, and who did not seem to be suspicious people, he did not return at once to La Junta but wandered for ten moons among different nations. When he was ready to return he learned that some of his people had been killed by "the Satapayogliglas, Sisimbles, and other Indian nations... because they would not join with them against the Spaniards, and he had to go out with a body of men in search of the said nations, with whom he has had and is still having wars .... For [this] reason he would not have come so soon to [Parral] if it had not been that he went to the pueblo of San Antonio [de Julimes] in search of the governor of the Julimes, in order to ask him to go to La Junta de los Ríos and aid him with four or five hundred of his own Indians against the said nations...." Sabeata said that he had not been to El Paso, which was a long trip and through enemy territory. He was described in this testimony as the governor of the Cibola and Jumano Indians (Hackett 1926:285–89).

For ten turbulent years Sabeata appeared in the records as the leader of the Jumanos and associated groups. Summarized, his travels during the decade of 1682–1692 are enlightening as to the nomadic life of the Jumanos

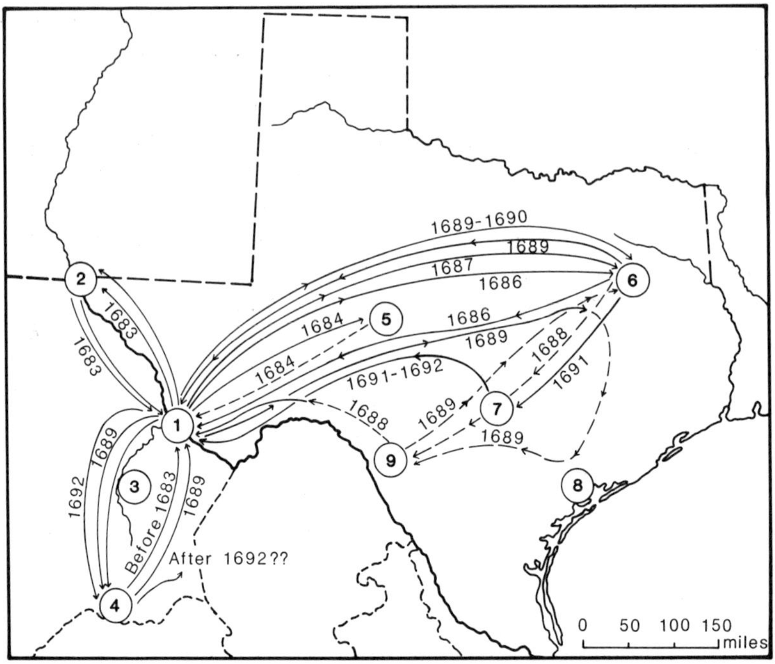

Figure 2. Travels of the Jumanos, 1683–1692. Lines of travel indicated are diagrammatic only. **1** La Junta; **2** El Paso del Norte; **3** San Antonio de Julimes; **4** Parral; **5** "Rio Nueces"; **6** Tejas or Hasinai villages; **7** Rancherias on the Guadalupe River near New Braunfels; **8** La Salle's fort on the Garcitas River; **9** Rancherias of the "Sierra" (probably the Anacacho Mountains).

(Fig. 2). Sabeata made two round-trips between La Junta and El Paso in 1683, and he had made at least one trip to Parral prior to this date, because he stated that he had been baptized there (Hackett 1931:137). In 1684 he led the Mendoza expedition to the Rio Nueces. It is assumed that he returned to La Junta the following winter, but we have no record of this. The rebellion that broke out among the Suma Indians along the Rio Grande above La Junta before Mendoza's return to El Paso may have been in part inspired by Sabeata, who was sent away in anger by Mendoza. The Tejas told Douay that their warriors had been with the Jumanos fighting the Spaniards. This was in the spring or summer of 1686; two years previous two Tejas Indians had been with Sabeata at La Junta and had accompanied him to the Rio Nueces, and shortly thereafter the Suma revolt occurred. Previously the Jumanos had been continuously at peace with the Spaniards, suggesting that the Suma outbreak was the occasion referred to by the Tejas. Furthermore, it may be confidently assumed that the "Chouman ambassadors" at the Tejas towns in 1687 who told Douay in such detail of the Spanish settlements and habits included Sabeata, in view of other data regarding his behavior. Likewise, the group of Jumano-Cibolas who asked the priests at La Junta for a letter to give to the French in east Texas in 1687 were followers of Sabeata, if not including Sabeata himself, and were presumably starting out for the Tejas towns at that time. We know from the Parral testimonies that Sabeata was among the Tejas in 1687 or 1688, and that he was bringing a Frenchman with him on his return to La Junta. Reasons for believing that Sabeata was at Anacacho Mountain in 1688 are discussed in the next chapter.

Later in the same year, apparently in November, he was, by his own statement, at La Junta. Even later that year, or more probably in the late winter of 1688, he left La Junta, traveled until he reached the outlying Tejas towns, then south "almost to the sea" near the French fort, and to the "Indians of the Sierra," then back to the Tejas towns, from where he returned to La Junta, meeting Retana on the Pecos River early in March, 1689. He then went to Parral to testify, his second recorded trip there. Presumably he returned to La Junta, and from there went to the Tejas towns either later in the same year or the following year, since the letter given him by the Spanish missionaries among the Tejas was dated September 4, 1690 (Hackett 1926:285–89).

After 1692 Sabeata does not again appear in the records, nor do we have any further records of Jumanos at Parral. In 1692, Sabeata declared that he was more than fifty years of age. If even approximately true, he was well advanced in years for the active leader of such a wandering group as the Jumanos. It is perhaps significant that the disappearance of this wily and forceful leader coincides with the disappearance of the Jumanos as an important group, and their apparent absorption by their old enemies, the Apaches, whom Sabeata had so valiantly fought. Nor, after 1692, do we have any further records of Jumanos who can be identified with certainty as the Jumanos whose history we have been tracing. In the spring and summer of 1693, Gregorio Salinas traveled from Monclova to the missions of the Tejas country and returned again to Coahuila. He reported seeing the "Jumanes" on the route, in all probability the main Jumano group or the Eagle Pass division.[21]

5

The Eagle Pass Jumanos

During the period just discussed, from 1675 to 1693, references were frequently made to a Jumano group near the Rio Grande from the vicinity of the Devils River south to near Eagle Pass and below the Rio Grande in Coahuila. This group may have been a detached division of the Jumanos, but there is a possibility that it may have been an entirely different and unrelated group. A brief outline of the references to this group is given below.

In 1675, at the post of San Ysidro north of the Rio Grande above Eagle Pass and apparently east of the Pecos River near the "Sierra Dacate," (probably, as Bolton [1916:287] points out, the present Anacacho Mountains) and probably on the Devils River above Del Rio, Fernando del Bosque, Fray Juan Larios, and Fray Buenaventura were visited by a group of Indians, including the Xomans (Jumanos?), the Teroodans (Tercodames?), the Teanames, and the Teimamar. These Indians said they were "heathens" and had never seen the Spaniards. This would be entirely possible at this early date if the Jumanos concerned had been a local division of the tribe which had not visited the north Mexican settlements. They said that they wished to be baptized and settle down in pueblos. Perhaps significantly, the Spaniards noted that among the Indians of the region were the Catujanes, Tilijaes, Apes, and Pachaques (Bolton 1916: 281–309). It will be recalled that as far back as 1630 Benavides noted the Iapes, possibly the Apes described here, were neighbors of the Jumanos proper (see Chapter 3).

In 1688 the Jumanos were mentioned in Coahuila in connection with the Teocodames (Tercodames), who apparently lived in the vicinity of Eagle Pass on the Rio Grande. Don Dieguillo, Indian leader of the Colorados,

Cabezas, and Tobozos, with others in revolt at that time attempted to enlist the support of these Jumanos.[1] Judging from the associated tribes and the general location, this would seem to have been the "Xoman" group mentioned in the Bosque-Larios records. Also in 1688, a messenger sent by Captain Diego Ramón to call the Tercodames, Herbiapames, and Jumanos to the Nadadores mission stated that he had been to the Jumanos and that they reported that, some time before, the French had come there with some of the Tejas Indians and that all had gone in friendship to make an attack on the Apaches, after which the French returned to their town.[2] Again, the association of the Jumanos with the Tercodames indicated that they were the same group as that previously noted above in the Eagle Pass neighborhood. Their associations with the French and the Tejas, and their warlike relations with the Apaches suggest that they may have been a branch of the Jumanos proper.

In the same year, Massanet reported that Juan, captain of the same Pacpul nation, had been sent to a rancheria of Indians in the Sacatsol Mountains—the Dacate Mountains of the Bosque-Larios expedition—20 leagues beyond the Rio Grande from Coahuila and 60 leagues from the San Salvador mission. A Frenchman, a deserter from La Salle's party, was reported to be living with the Indians there. Juan went to the rancheria, which was occupied by many nations, including the "Mescales, Yoricas, Chomenes, Machomenes, Sampanales, Paquachiams, Tilpayay, [and] Apis," and persuaded the Frenchman to leave. The Spaniards, on seeing the Frenchman, remarked that he was "painted like the Indians" (Bolton 1916:356–87). Here we have an additional evidence that the Jumanos of the Eagle Pass-Devils River region may have been the true Jumanos. Not only were they associated with the Apis (Apes?), as previously noted, but in addition they had with them one of the French deserters. Referring back to the Parral testimonies, it will be noted that in 1688, the year in question here, it was reported in La Junta that the Jumanos proper were en route to La Junta with a Frenchman from La Salle's party (see Chapter 4). When they actually arrived, however, the Frenchman was not with them; they brought only French documents to prove their story. Obviously the Jumanos who lost a Frenchman at the Dacate Mountains in 1688 could be the Jumanos who in the same year sent word to La Junta that they were coming with such a Frenchman, only to appear without him.

In 1689 the De León expedition halted at a rancheria of "Hapes, Jumenes, Xiabu, [and] Mescale" Indians, with others, located some four leagues south of the Rio Grande near modern Eagle Pass. This was the same group as that found at the Dacate Mountains the previous year, because the Frenchman who had been with them then was sent forward as an envoy on this occasion, and was received by them with great joy. A hut was prepared for him "covered with buffalo hides" before which was "driven a stake, four *varas* high, on which were fastened sixteen heads of Indians, their enemies, whom they had killed" (Bolton 1916:389). There were 85 huts in this camp, and 490 Indians altogether, of the joined nations. Some of these were armed while others were not. The Spaniards distributed cotton garments, blankets, beads, rosaries, knives, and arms among them.

The De León expedition of 1690 noted, in about this same location, five leagues south of the Rio Grande, "the Indians of The Frenchman" to whom they gave tobacco and clothing (Bolton 1916:406). This apparently was the same group noted in 1689.

Again, in 1691, the Teran-Massanet expedition found in this same region from five to ten leagues south of the Rio Grande, Indians of the Mescaleros, Yoricas, "Chome,"[3] Parchacas, Alachome, and Pamais tribes. Massanet noted that

> all these tribes live between the Rio del Norte and the Sabinas. They are not located in any definite place but always roam about hunting buffaloes and searching for what the country affords. They do not plant crops nor do they do anything that resembles work.[4]

Although this group, judging from its location and associated tribes, was the Jumano group previously noted in this area, it was not the Jumano group under the direct leadership of Juan Sabeata, because this group was found several days later by the same expedition on the Guadalupe River some distance north of the Rio Grande.

In general, the Jumanos (Chome, Chomanes, Jumanes, etc.) of the Eagle Pass-Devils River region seem to be a division of Jumanos as far as the historical evidence is concerned. This conclusion is based on the evidence already submitted: their association with the Ape Indians; their friendly relations with the French and the Tejas; their possession of the French deserter; and their relations with the Pacpuls. On the other hand, several items would seem to indicate that they represented at most only a distant branch of the main group. Their associations were slightly different; the Cibolas are not mentioned in their company, and instead they seem firm friends and allies of the Tercodames, the Mescales, and others, who were rarely encountered with the Jumanos under Sabeata. Juan Sabeata was not mentioned by name in connection with this group, although it is to be inferred from the affair of the Frenchman that he was associated with them at times. Also, in 1675 the group said that they were heathen and had not seen Spaniards, while evidence already presented would tend to show that the Spaniards were in constant touch with the Jumanos of the "Rio Nueces" during this period. The range of this particular group seems to have been from the present-day Nueces River (not the Rio Nueces/Concho of other accounts) on the east, the Devils River on the north, to the Rio Savanas of Coahuila on the southwest, and the Tercodame territory around Eagle Pass on the southeast. Thus, their range was contiguous with the Sabeata-Jumano range from the Guadalupe River to La Junta. If they were actually true Jumanos they must have remained more or less permanently on the buffalo hunt in that region, and perhaps were only nominally attached to the Jumanos under Sabeata, if at all. The archaeological evidence would seem to indicate that the Eagle Pass Jumanos were not the same as the Jumanos of Juan Sabeata.

6

The Jumanos

1694–1771

After abandonment of Texas by the Spaniards in 1693 and following its reoccupation in 1716, the Jumanos seem to have remained in their old range but to have changed their political affiliations, slowly shifting from a deadly enmity toward the Apaches to becoming their friends and allies and eventually coming to be known themselves as "Apaches Jumanes." During the same period they became enemies of most of their old friends, including the Tejas. Bolton (1911:79–86) has presented a detailed account of this change citing many references in regard to it. Since it adds little to our primary discussion, only an abbreviated paraphrase of Bolton's account is given here.[1]

From 1693 to 1700 the Jumanos continued as enemies of the Apaches, according to the statement of the Spaniard Joseph de Urrutia, who said that he led many nations in battle against the Apaches, including the Jumanos and the Pelones. In 1706 a Jumano Indian at Monclova gave information obtained from a Timamar Indian; judging from this association, the Eagle Pass Jumanos were involved but no data regarding affiliations with the Apaches were given. In 1716, however, Domingo de Ramón noted the Jumanos, the Apaches, and the Chanas were enemies of the Tejas Indians. From 1721–1722 a Coahuila Indian served as a slave to the Tobosos and the Jumanos; the latter, he stated, accompanied the Spanish missionaries in their travels among the Tobosos, who, it is known, were either themselves Apaches or closely affiliated with them. In 1731 an Apache captive at San Antonio spoke of some discarded arrows as belonging to Apaches, Jumanos, and Pelones, all of whom were warlike and numerous, terrorizing the region and conquering all other nations. The following year, 1732, Bustillo y Zevallos, governor of Texas, attacked a rancheria of Apaches, Ypandas (Pelones?), Yxandes, and Chentis; the captives who were taken stated that the main group was a short distance north and west, the rancheria itself containing none "of the Jumanes Nation . . . which is [known to be] very numerous and which . . . joins with that of the Apaches to come and make war" on the Spaniards. Again, in 1732 and 1734 references were made to "Apaches, Pelones, Jumanas, Chenttis," and to "Apaches, Pelon, and Xumanes" as enemies of the Spaniards.

After 1732 the Jumanos gradually came to be regarded not only as allies of the Apaches but as Apaches themselves. The same Joseph de Urrutia, captain at San Antonio, stated that the Jumanos apparently "have now incorporated themselves in the said Apaches, which to me is very strange, because in that time [1693–1700], when I lived among them, they were declared enemies" (Bolton 1911:82). In 1746, Bustillo wrote of the continual war carried on with, among others, the "Apaches Jumanes, who, crossing the deserts of the province of Coahuila, pass to the Kingdom and to the neighborhood of Saltillo"; and further regarding Coahuila, "The arms of the capital of this province . . . restrain the Nations of the Apaches Jumanes, who are immediately on the other side of the Rio Grande, and at times on this side." Finally, in 1773, Alexo. de la Garza Falcón wrote from the presidio of San Saba regarding the

> imminent danger in which [the presidio] now stands of being attacked by the barbarous, hostile nations of Indians, Apaches, Farones, Natages, Mescaleros, Jumanes, Lipanes, and other frontier nations allied with them, both on account of the continual robberies and murders which they commit [in] this neighborhood, and because there are now at a distance of ten leagues from this *Presidio* about 3,000 of said nations . . . who . . . having come out victorious from an encounter which they had with the Comanches and Taguaias [Taovayas], gathered to celebrate the victory and eat some of the Comanche and Taguaias prisoners whom they captured. [Bolton 1911:83–84]

According to Bolton, this is the only reference after 1750 to a group which can be identified with the southern Jumanos (the true Jumanos).

The Jumanos of 1693 and 1706 were probably the Jumanos proper, since their range, political affiliations, and name remained the same; but the Jumanos of 1716–1771 who were friends, allies, and perhaps a subdivision of the Apaches, and enemies of the Tejas and Spaniards, can be identified with earlier Jumanos, enemies of the Apaches and friends of the Tejas and Spaniards only by the continuity of tribal name and range. In spite of this it seems probable that this group was the true Jumanos. Joseph de Urrutia, already quoted, seemed to believe so when he remarked on the strangeness of the change. There is also another bit of indirect evidence which Bolton did not mention.

While at La Junta in 1716 for the purpose of re-establishing the missions there, Don Juan Antonio de Trasviña Retís wrote as follows:

> I spent the entire day in said pueblo [San Francisco, at the junction of the rivers]... and sent a call to the governors and to the oldest and most experienced Indians, who, being all assembled, I questioned them again and again through the interpreter, General Antonio de la Cruz [Governor of the Julimes, and a native of La Junta], regarding the information about the Colorado River as well as the Pearl Sea or Pearl Lake, which was mentioned in a letter to Colonel... Masoni by Reverend Father Andrés Ramirez as having been reported by an Apache Indian whom he baptized and who reported said lake to be six days' travel from La Junta. The most experienced Indians replied that no one from those pueblos had ever been there and that they had heard of it only from the said Apache, whom they had taken to be their friend. He promised them that when teaching missionaries should come to these pueblos, he would bring all the people of his rancheria, which are about sixty families above and below La Junta so that they should all be catechized and baptized. Failure to notify the said Apache... was due to knowledge that there was smallpox on his rancheria. When he comes, as he is in the habit of doing, they will send him to me with an interpreter so that I may question him.... Likewise I asked how far it is from this place to Coahuila but no one could tell me because they had not been over the country. [Reindorp 1938:17–18]

Later, after returning to San Francisco de Cuellar, Trasviña added a further note in this regard:

> Captain Don Pedro gave me news that the Apache Indian who was baptized by Father Fray Andrés Ramirez and who named Don Antonio de la Cruz, the General of Julimes Pueblo of La Junta de los Rios for his godfather came [to that place] for he had learned that I had conducted the fathers there. But he arrived too late. He, therefore, told the Indians of La Junta to advise me that he would come to this Real as soon as he returns from the Colorado River, where he went to get information for me about that and other places. [Reindorp 1938:24]

No mention of the Jumanos at La Junta occurs in Trasviña's account, although all the other groups noted there in 1683–1684 were listed. The Cibolas were noted as having joined the Polacmes at Guadalupe pueblo, which was "well built with two plazas dividing the two nations which are united for mutual defense from the enemies that have attacked them from time to time because [they] did not care to admit the assemblies of these hostile Indians to go with them up into the mountains" (Reindorp 1938:17).

The groups which are listed had not only the same names but the same culture, both archaeologically and historically, as those of La Junta in 1683 and as the earlier Patarabueyes of 1581–1583 and can be regarded as one group. The "Apaches," with their rancherias near La Junta, their friendly visits there for baptism and probably for trade, their travels to the Colorado River and "Pearl Lake," obviously the Pearl River, a branch of the "Rio Nueces" of the seventeenth century accounts, and their intimate relations with the Julimes, as well as their willingness to travel and obtain information for the Spaniards stood in the same relation to the La Junta settlements as had the Jumanos in the previous century. Since the Jumanos were not again mentioned at La Junta,[2] and since they were elsewhere in their former range coming to be known as allies of the Apaches, if not Apaches themselves, and since Apaches had not previously been noted at

La Junta, it seems highly probable that the "Apaches" of the 1716 accounts were actually Jumanos. As a corollary, the case for the identification of the Apaches-Jumanes with the earlier Jumanos is considerably strengthened.

In general, the coincidence of the appearance of the Jumanos as allies of the Apaches and then as Apaches-Jumanes immediately following the last references to the true Jumanos, and as occupants of the same region, with the same range, and with the same relation with the Patarabueyes of La Junta, is so close as to render the identification of Jumanos as Apaches-Jumanes reasonably conclusive. Thus, we have traced the history of the Jumano nation fairly continuously from 1583 to 1771 over a territory ranging from La Junta to the Colorado River and southwestward to the Gulf Coast and the Rio Savanas of Coahuila, and, as visitors, as far away from home as the Tejas towns in east Texas, Isleta pueblo in New Mexico, El Paso, Parral, and Monclova. After fighting the Apaches for over a century, the Jumanos were finally forced or enticed into alliance with them and eventually were absorbed into the Apache nation.

The culture of the Jumanos is poorly known despite the many references to the group over a period of nearly two centuries. A complete trait list is given in Chapter 15. In making this list, as well as in the historical discussions presented above, only those references have been used that apply to groups identifiable with some assurance as the Jumanos proper; all references to groups obviously so termed because of their *rayado* decoration, such as the Taovayas, the Wichita proper, the Pawnee, the Havasupai, and to "Jumano" groups of dubious affiliation, have been omitted. The culture of the Patarabueyes, as well as references to them in documentary sources, has likewise been omitted since they were obviously a distinct group, though erroneously called Jumanos by Espejo. In order to demonstrate this distinction, as well as to present the true facts of Jumano-Patarabueye relationship at La Junta, it will be necessary to trace the parallel but distinct development of Patarabueye culture and history.

Part III

Historical Data: The Patarabueyes

7

The Patarabueyes
1535–1583

The crux of the entire Jumano problem lies in the correct identification of a series of related Indian groups that the sixteenth-century Spanish explorers found dwelling along the lower Conchos River of Chihuahua for a few leagues above its junction with the Rio Grande at La Junta and a similar distance above and below the junction on the latter stream. These Indians lived in organized villages of permanent houses, and cultivated maize and beans. Several loosely federated ethnic groups forming a more or less homogeneous cultural unit were represented. They were called, collectively, "Patarabueyes" by the early explorers,[1] and are so termed throughout this study.

Generally, the Patarabueyes have been confused with the Jumanos, and the ample cultural data pertaining to the former usually have been assigned gratuitously to the latter. This error has long created confusion, especially among archaeologists. Thus, Gladwin wrote in his reconstruction of Chihuahuan archaeological history, "Spanish identification of the Jumano, of Caddoan stock, with the makers of red-on-brown pottery and polished redware gives further confirmation of the link between Caddoan and Mogollon" (Gladwin, in Sayles 1936:101). Actually, the Patarabueyes, not the Jumanos, were the makers of the red-on-brown pottery in question, and the Jumanos may or may not have been of Caddoan stock. Some workers, notably Bandelier and Sauer, noted the discrepancy and attempted an explanation. Bandelier correctly surmised that the Patarabueyes, or the Julimes, as the principal Patarabueye group was termed after the sixteenth century, and the Jumanos lived together at La Junta, but were actually separate groups (Bandelier 1890). Sauer did not recognize the distinction in the sixteenth century between Jumanos and Patarabueyes, and minimized the Jumano influence at La Junta in the seventeenth century. He concluded therefore that the Jumanos had occupied La Junta at the beginning of the historic period but were dispossessed and driven eastward in the seventeenth century by the expansion of the Julimes and other Conchos tribes down the Conchos River (Sauer 1934).

It will be shown that the La Junta group called the Patarabueyes by Luxán in 1582 lived in the same villages and had the same culture as the Conchos-speaking Julimes and related tribes of the seventeenth and eighteenth centuries, and that throughout their history they were ethnically distinct from the Jumanos whose history we have traced in detail in the previous chapters. Ample historical and archaeological data are available for this purpose; in this chapter only the historical data are utilized.

It is remotely possible that Cabeza de Vaca and his companions visited the Patarabueye villages of La Junta in 1535, but the evidence is somewhat contradictory.

After traversing an expanse of dry and rugged mountains, de Vaca and his companions halted on "certain plains at the base of the mountains, where people came to meet [them] from a great distance" (Hodge 1907:100). These Indians told the Spaniards that the country to the north was lacking in water and food, and no people were to be found except at a great distance, and that toward the west inhabitants were far away.[2] The people toward the west were their enemies. Reluctantly the Indians sent two women to the people in the west, one a captive taken from them previously. After several days the women returned "and said they had found very few people; nearly all had gone for cattle, being then in the season." The Indians and Spaniards traveled three days and then Estevanico and Castillo took the two women as guides and went on six leagues ahead, where they were later joined by de Vaca. "She that was the captive led them to the river which ran between some ridges, where was a town at which her father lived; and these habitations were the first seen, having the appearance and structure of houses" (Hodge 1907:102).[3]

The people of the town were not only enemies of the previous group, but they also spoke a different language. These town-dwelling Indians may have been the Patarabueyes. They were called the "People of the Cows" by the Spaniards. The country was well settled, and there were several towns scattered along the river, which apparently ran almost west and east at this point. Farther up the same river, the route followed by the Spaniards on leaving, were other peoples who were their enemies but who spoke the same language, and who lacked food but had bison skins, and cotton mantles. To the west lived people who had much maize, and to the north "along that river" for over 50 leagues they went to kill bison. It is probable that this was not the same river on which the settlements were located, but one to the north, possibly the Pecos, because the Spaniards followed the river of the settlements westwardly.

The People of the Cows were active, strong people who understood the Spaniards' questions easily and answered them intelligently. The women were dressed in deerskins. Most of the men wore nothing, with the exception of the aged who were no longer capable of fighting. They received the Spaniards in their houses, seated with their faces to the wall, their hair dropped before their lowered faces, and all "their property placed in a heap in the middle of the house" (Hodge 1907:103). Festivities were held when the Spaniards arrived and houses had been readied for their occupancy.

These Indians lived by cultivating beans and calabashes, and normally maize, although a two-year drought had destroyed their supplies and prevented them from successfully planting more. They begged the Spaniards to ask the sky to rain. They had blankets of bison skin, water gourds, wooden tongs, and other things. Their method of cooking, by stone boiling, was new and strange to the Spaniards, who said

> Not having discovered the use of pipkins [Ellos no alcan con ollas] to boil what they would eat, they fill the half of a large calabash with water, and throw on the fire many stones of such as are most convenient and readily take the heat. When hot, they are taken up with tongs of sticks and dropped into the calabash until the water in it boils from the fervor of the stones. Then whatever is to be cooked is put in, and until it is done they continue taking out cooled stones and throwing in hot ones. Thus they boil their food. [Hodge 1907:105]

The Bandelier (1905:154) translation gives this somewhat differently, stating, "They have no pots. In order to cook their food they fill a middle-sized gourd with water. . . . "

If we accept the Bandelier translation, or possibly even following the Hodge edition, we are faced with a curious contradiction. The description of the culture of the People of the Cows, of their land, the locations of other groups and of the bison, together with the apparent route of the de Vaca expedition, makes it seem possible that the People of the Cows were the Patarabueyes; in fact, the latter group in 1582 informed the Espejo expedition that de Vaca and his companions had been there.[4] But if the People of the Cows had no pots, it seems impossible that they could have been the Patarabueyes, since the archaeological data indicate conclusively that the occupants of the La Junta towns had pottery well back into prehistoric times, probably as early as A.D. 1200. True, they had very small amounts of pottery in prehistoric times, but it seems impossible that de Vaca could have failed to observe such pottery as they did have. Possibly de Vaca has confused two distinct groups, and the People of the Cows were Patarabueyes, but there is no assurance of the validity of such an interpretation.

Between 1535 and 1582 the Patarabueyes do not appear in the Spanish documentary sources to which I have had access. Following the founding of the mining camp of Santa Barbara in southern Chihuahua about 1563, however, the Patarabueyes were subjected to visits by Spanish slave-raiding parties.[5] In 1582 the Rodríguez expedition followed the Conchos River to La Junta and continued up the Rio Grande into New Mexico, returning by the same route later in the year. The Gallegos account of this expedition furnishes the first detailed account of the Patarabueyes and their culture (Hammond and Rey 1927:14–21). Below the rancherias of the Conchos Indians and just above Cuchillo Parado[6] the explorers came to the Cabris nation, possibly the Julimes Indians of later expeditions. According to the Spaniards, the Cabris spoke a language different from that of the leading Patarabueye group, the Amotomancos, but both groups were able to understand one another, suggesting that the linguistic difference was a dialectic one. Luxán calls this group the Passaguates, and notes that they were "friends of the Conchos and Patarabueyes, because they speak all three languages" (Hammond and Rey 1929:54). This seems to substantiate the similarity between Patarabueye and Cabris, and to class both languages with the Conchos; this is borne out by later accounts of the same peoples. However, bilingualism, or even trilingualism, is not unknown among Indian groups. The Cabris appear quite similar in culture to the Patarabueyes and should be classed with them rather than with the Conchos farther upstream. According to Gallegos, the Cabris were tall, handsome, spirited, active, and intelligent and "their faces, arms and bodies are striped with pleasing lines. [They] are cleaner and more modest than the Concha." They went naked and wore their hair "in the shape of skull caps." They cultivated beans and calabashes, and also used ground mesquite, prickly pears, and mushrooms as food the year around. They described the Pueblo Indians, of whom they had heard. At this time they were apparently at war with the Patarabueyes who lived farther downstream (Hammond and Rey 1927:14).

Below Cuchillo Parado were found the Amotomancos.[7] The people were "clean, handsome, and warlike, the best featured . . . encountered." They were "striped people and very merry." They wore no clothes, but lived in permanent houses. Gallegos wrote:

> These houses resemble those of the Mexicans, except that they are made of paling. They build them square. They put up the bases and upon these they place timbers, the thickness of a man's thigh. Then they add the pales, and plaster them with mud. Close to them they have their granaries built of willow, after the fashion of the Mexicans, where they keep their provisions and their harvest of mesquite and other things. [Hammond and Rey 1927:18]

In one pueblo there were "eight large square houses inhabited by many people, over three hundred persons in number." The Indians stood on top of these houses when the Spaniards arrived and showed great merriment at the sight of the explorers.

They cultivated some corn, and beans and calabashes in quantity. Their "natural food" was mushrooms,[8] and they also had ground mesquite and prickly pears. They called water "abad," corn "teoy," and beans "ayaguate." They had "Turkish bows" and arrows, and cowhide shields, all very well made, and possessed many tanned bison skins. They had a form of drum made by attaching skins to a "vessel," in the form of a tambourine. The mention of the "vessel" is the nearest approach to a note on the presence of pottery at La Junta in the documentary sources. The La Junta pottery must have been particularly rare or unimpressive in appearance. On this drum they produced a dance rhythm

> resembling negroes' dances . . . they rise and perform their dances to the rhythm of the music like merry-andrews. They raise their hands toward the sun and sing a dance tune in their language, 'ayia canima.' They do this with much compass and harmony, in such a way that although there are three hundred men in a dance, it seems as if it were being sung and danced by one only, due to the good harmony and measure with which they do it. [Hammond and Rey 1927:21]

The Amotomancos had deer skins and feathers. One Indian had a piece of copper, called "porba," suspended around his neck with cotton threads and another had a copper sleigh bell. They said they obtained these items from the west. Others wore white and colored coral, "although not of fine quality," and turquoises suspended from the nose. The coral came from the sea "as they pointed that way." They also "saw another Indian who brought us an iron bar about three yards long and shaped like those possessed by the Mexican Indians." This they said came from the direction "where . . . the clothed and settled people were located" (the Pueblo Indians?).

The Spaniards talked with old Indians who seemed to be caciques of that land. The other Indians obeyed one such cacique "to such an extent that they carried a seat that he could sit down. It consisted of a very large tanned cowhide." The old men indicated that the land occupied by people of their tongue extended over 100 leagues. Farther up the Rio Grande was another nation and language, people who were their enemies (the Mansos near and above El Paso?). They said that thirteen days upstream were many clothed people, presumably the Pueblo Indians, and when asked whether they had been there they replied that they had not, but that they had heard about it long ago from the people who killed the cattle and that they considered it very certain. The Indians told the Spaniards that a long time ago four Christians had passed through. Gallegos is certain from the description that this referred to the party of Alvar Nuñez Cabeza de Vaca. In general the Amotomancos reacted very favorably to the Spaniards, gave them many presents, and accompanied them as guides to the end of their territory.

Obregón's history of 1584, although a secondary source and in many ways not fully trustworthy, adds a few items of Patarabueye culture to the list just given. Spears and clubs are listed among the Patarabueye weapons, maguey among their foods. Obregón states that they were weavers of cloth. They also fished. Their bison skins were obtained by trade. They gave the Spaniards considerable information about the Pueblo Indians. There were some two thousand Indians in the La Junta vicinity. According to Obregón they worshipped the sun and made many faces and signs toward the sky to denote their respect. Obregón describes the Patarabueye houses as "terraced houses" (Hammmond and Rey 1928:273–82).[9]

In 1582, following the return of the Rodríguez expedition, the Espejo expedition entered New Mexico by the same route used by the earlier group. Various short summaries of the events of the trip written by Espejo and a journal of the *entrada* kept by Diego Pérez de Luxán are the best sources for Patarabueye data furnished by this expedition. These accounts verify the descriptions given by the historians of the Rodríguez expedition and supply many additional items.

Luxán's diary supplies the following data (Hammond and Rey 1929). At the Cuchillo Parado boundary of the La Junta country lived the Passaguates, while along the Rio Conchos and Rio Grande lived the Otomoacos. At the junction of the two rivers they found the Abriache Indians. The Abriaches and Otomoacos were Patarabueye groups; the Passaguates, on the other hand, appear to have been transitional between Patarabueyes and Conchos, and spoke both languages, as well as their own.

The Spaniards visited three principal pueblos and many rancherias along the two rivers, and noted that there were many others. These pueblos were Santo Tomás of the Abriache nation, San Juan Evangelista, and Santiago (see Map). Santo Tomás was located on a high mesa, less than a mile from the junction of the rivers, west of the Rio Conchos and south of the Rio Grande. In the late seventeenth century it was renamed San Francisco, a name which it has borne to this day. A cursory archaeological inspection indicated that this pueblo was first established sometime prior to A.D. 1400. San Juan Evangelista was not noted in the seventeenth century accounts and from archaeological evidence appears to have been deserted early in the historic period. It has been partially excavated by the author. It is located on a high mesa about a mile and a half due north of the river junction and some five miles northwest of Presidio, Texas, almost beside the Presidio-Candelaria highway. Santiago pueblo was renamed Nuestra Señora de Guadalupe of the Palacme and Cibola nations in the following century, and bore that name until its abandonment shortly before the beginning of the nineteenth century. Its ruins lie on the edge of the first terrace of the Rio Grande above the floodplain, on the north bank some five miles below the junction, and the edge of the modern town of New Presidio, Texas. A large portion of this ruin was excavated by Donald J. Lehmer and the author. It was founded, in all probability, sometime in the thirteenth century and was well populated throughout its subsequent occupation.

Santo Tomás had a population of about six hundred people, and was ruled by the cacique Baij Sibiye. San Juan Evangelista had a "suburb" at the foot of the mesa, while the main pueblo on the mesa was made up of many flat-roofed houses, with a neatly kept plaza (Plate I, and Figs. 3–9).

> The Indians of this city are all farmers, as the river is very appropriate for it, because it forms many damp islands and bays. And even though they live in the pueblos they have flat-roofed houses in their fields where they reside during harvest time. [Hammond and Rey 1929:62]

Its cacique was Casica Moyo. Santiago was the largest of all the pueblos. It was ruled by the cacique Q. Bisise, "whom all other caciques respected."

These flat-roofed houses in the fields, as described at the rancheria called San Bernardino five leagues above La Junta, were semi-pithouses, "half under and half above the ground."

As to the Patarabueye costume, Luxán says:

> These people are naked and have their privy parts uncovered. They cover themselves with well tanned skins of the [bison]. These hides they tan and soften by beating them with stones until they are soft. . . . The women wear some sort of tanned deerskin bodices resembling scapularies which cover their breasts, and other tanned deerskins as skirts, carrying as cloaks tanned skins of the cattle. These people wear their hair long and tied to the head. The men have their hair cut very short, up to the middle of their heads, and from there up they leave it two fingers long and curl it with minimum paint in such a way that it resembles a small cap. They leave on the crown a large lock of hair to which they fasten feathers of white and black birds such as geese, cranes, and sparrow-hawks. [Hammond and Rey 1929:57–58]

Elsewhere Luxán mentions "adornments in the shape of feather caps"; "ornaments like bonnets with colored feathers which they said they obtained from the direction of the sea"; "shawls"; and "native blankets."

The Patarabueyes cultivated maize, beans, and calabashes, and had "vegetables" and much mescal. They ate fish[10] and had bison meat. Luxán noted that they "ordinarily go for the meat and skins where [the bison] roam, which is about thirty leagues from this province." They used bows and arrows in fighting and hunting. These bows were the best the Spaniards had ever seen: "The bows are Turkish, all reinforced and very strong, and the strings are made from the sinews of the buffalo."

The Patarabueyes greeted the Spaniards with great joy, gave them gifts, and held celebrations in their honor. In all the pueblos the people met them "with music similar to that of the flute but made with their mouths." Luxán describes their celebrations: "On this night they carried on great dances and rejoicing. They made music by beating their hands while sitting around a big fire. They sing, and in time with the singing they dance, a few rising from one side and others from the opposite, performing their dances two, four, and eight at a time" (Hammond and Rey 1929:67). This is quite similar to the dance described by Gallegos. In both cases the Spaniards were near the northern boundary of the Patarabueyes when these dances were performed for them.

While the Spaniards were at Santiago pueblo and "in all the others" they were told "how Cabeza de Vaca and his two companions and a negro had been there." In most of the pueblos they found crosses that had been erected by the Rodríguez expedition.

Several days' travel up the Rio Grande the Spaniards came to another nation, the Caguates. "An old cacique from the Caguates nation named Guaxi came to the place. He was a grandfather of Pedro, the [Patarabueye] interpreter.... They [were] friendly and intermarried with the Otomoacos and almost [had] the same language." There were more than three hundred Caguate Indians. They performed dances for the Spaniards. They had made a stable for a horse lost by the Rodríguez party and gave it the best of care, feeding it and talking to it "as if it were a person."[11]

Espejo's own account of the expedition (translated in Bolton 1916) adds a few items worthy of note. He states that the Passaguates ("Pazaguates") had "rancherias, huts, and food like the Conchos." Patarabueye was another name for the Jumano Indians, according to Bolton (1916:172).[12] He claims there were five pueblos with more than ten thousand Indians, and flat-roofed houses, low and well arranged into pueblos. They were settled along the Rio Grande "for a distance of twelve days' journey. Some of them [had] flat-roofed houses, and others [lived] in grass huts." The people were very large and had "their faces streaked." In addition to prickly pear and the plant foods mentioned by Luxán, they had "game of foot and wing, and fish of many kinds from the two rivers." The Patarabueyes made moccasins of bison hide. They pointed to the heavens with respect, saying "Apalito," which Espejo says was their word for God. The Spaniards gave the Patarabueyes beads, hats, and other things.

Espejo gives a most interesting account of the group up river from La Junta which Luxán identified as the Caguate nation, closely related to the Patarabueyes:

> They brought us many things made of feathers of different colors, and some small cottom *mantas,* striped with blue and white, like some of those they bring from China; and they gave us to understand by signs that another nation that adjoined theirs, towards the west,

> brought these things to barter with them for other goods which these [*sic*] had and which appeared from what they told us by signs to be dressed hides of cows and deer.... [Bolton 1916:174]

Obregón's account of the Espejo expedition (Hammond and Rey 1928:317–19) is merely a paraphrase of the Espejo account and adds no new items. He gives Patarabueyes as "Patazagueyes," and perpetuates Espejo's error in calling them Jumanos.

8

The Patarabueyes

1584–1694

There is no surviving evidence of any Spanish expedition that visited La Junta and the Patarabueye Indians between 1583 and 1659. The name Patarabueye appears only twice more in the documentary sources that I have seen. In 1595, Oñate's petition to the viceroy regarding the organization of his projected colonization of New Mexico contained the following item: "They must give me the Indians that are to be found in this City of Mexico of the nation Tataragueyes [*sic*], for they are the nearest to that province..." The viceroy's agreement said, "Let him be given the Indians who seem to be of that province..." (Hackett 1923:234–35). In March, 1598, Oñate wrote to the King from the Rio Conchos. He reported that Vicente de Zaldivar had been sent with sixteen men to search out a new route to the Rio Grande (near El Paso). He said, referring to Zaldivar, "He heard of and avoided the village of the hostile Pataragueyes Indians, leaving it forty leagues to one side, on the right hand" (Hackett 1923:397). It is probable that more or less hostile relations prevailed between Spaniard and Patarabueye during this period, occasioned by the slave hunting proclivities of the former.

The founding of Nuestra Señora de Guadalupe and associated missions near El Paso del Norte on the Rio Grande probably opened a new era for the La Junta pueblos. Nevertheless we hear of no actual expeditions to the region until a decade or so later. Sometime prior to 1671 Fray García de San Francisco, founder of the El Paso mission, visited La Junta, said mass, and promised to return again. Shortly thereafter a religious of the same order, Fray Juan de Sumesta, visited the La Junta pueblo nearest to El Paso, where he soon returned (Hughes 1935:330).[1] Menchero reports that missions were first established at La Junta in 1670, but his account sounds so nearly identical with that of the missionary expedition of Father Lopez in 1683 that it is in all probability a mistake (Hackett 1937:407–8).[2] During this period, however, it is known that Julimes Indians from La Junta visited Parral, in Chihuahua, to work in the mines and plantations there. On numerous occasions they asked unsuccessfully for missionaries to be sent to them at La Junta.

In Chapter 4 the visit of the Jumano and Julimes Indians to El Paso in 1683, their request for missionaries, and the resulting visit of Father Lopez and two other priests, followed by the Mendoza party, to La Junta has been described. Sabeata, the Jumano chieftain, had been sent to El Paso by the captains of six La Junta nations, chief among which was that of the Julimes. These captains were all Christians (Hackett 1931:137–38). When Lopez and his fellow priests reached the first of the La Junta nations they found a "large church of grass" with an altar made according to the specifications of the altar in the El Paso mission, "and so arranged as to enable him to say mass." Six leagues farther on "he found another church much larger and more carefully built .... There was also a house ... built for the minister to live in." Later seven other nations built churches of their own. All these nations were settled and planted "quantities of corn, wheat, beans, calabashes, watermelons, cantaloupes, and tobacco" (Hackett 1934:349–52).[3] Father Posadas, speaking of the Lopez-Mendoza expedition, notes that Lopez found at La Junta

> muchos indios Jumanes, Rayados, Oposmes, Poleaques y otros, y que algonos de ellos sembraban maiz, frijo, trigo, calabazas y otras semillas; y los indios de estas naciones van por sus tiempos a trabajar a las sementeras del dicho Real del Parral y a sus minas, que distan de dicho paraje cien leguas. [Posadas, in Duro 1882:56]

Mendoza's own account of the La Junta tribes is short:

> We arrived at this place, which was named La Nabidad en las Cruces [La Junta], because of the crosses possessed by the rancherias which were settled on both sides of the Rio del Norte. These rancherias are of people of the Julimes nation; they are versed in the Mexican language, and all sow maize and wheat. [Bolton 1916:325]

In the spring of 1684, a revolt broke out among the Manso Indians near El Paso. This quickly spread to the Sumas, Janos, and Apaches, and in the summer to the Julimes Indians at La Junta, and the Conchos Indians farther up the Rio Conchos. The Christian Indians, however, remained faithful to the Spaniards and conducted the La Junta priests safely to Parral, taking with them the sacred vessels and ornaments from the churches (Hughes 1914:357, 358, 388). Thus, the first missionary effort at La Junta ended temporarily after less than two years of operation.

The La Junta missions were again functioning by 1687, the Manso revolt having ended in 1685. In 1688 at San Pedro de Conchos, Fray Agustín de

Colina, identified as "president of the missions of La Junta de los Ríos, on the Río del Norte," testified regarding the reports of the French in Texas. He stated that "in the past year, 1687, the Cíbolos and Jumanos Indians asked his paternity for a letter to the [French].... [T]his year [1688], in the month of September, five Cíbolos Indians came to La Junta de los Ríos and visited the said padre..." (Hackett 1926:241–43). In 1688, Fray Colina, writing from San Pedro de Conchos, said that he had gone to the presidio of San Francisco to "give account... concerning the reasons and motives of the superiors for leaving that country [La Junta], where we were for a year and seven months," and later,

> the prelate finds himself obliged to withdraw us, for the reason that the Suma nation is in a tumult, and it was not easy to protect us otherwise. Besides this, even supposing there were no uprising, the departure of the poor Indians to work on the haciendas, under conditions not such as our lord, the king, wishes for their conservation, [is bad] on account of the most of them remaining outside without the minister knowing how to induce them to accept Christian teaching. [This state of affairs] only originates with the native lieutenants and governors, whose sole aim is to draw out the required number of people. Others remain a long time merely to collect the price of their labor... [Hackett 1926:247]

Fray Colina complains bitterly regarding the failure of the authorities to pay the La Junta Indians for their labors, attributing much of the Indian trouble experienced by the Spaniards to this policy. Apparently the missionaries again returned to La Junta in 1688, since Retana, prior to going to La Junta, sent messengers there to inform the Indians that the priests who were with them in their missions were returning with him. In 1694 the royal officials of Durango wrote that "in the region known as La Junta de los Ríos... there have been no minister teachers, nor does it appear in the books of this royal auditor's office that there has been in the past any payment made... of any sum designated as aid for a mission in that region. In fact there has been no such payment" (Hackett 1926:361).

Apparently, between 1688 and 1715 the La Junta pueblos were, at the most, *visitas* of the missions at San Antonio de Julimes and San Pedro de Conchos. During this period the Patarabueyes normally were friendly to the Spaniards and aided them in fighting other Indian tribes on several occasions. The Patarabueyes, at this time, included the Julimes, Oposmes, Puliques, Polacmes, Conejos, Cacalotes, Mesquites, Posalmes, and probably some Rayados, Jumanos, Cibolas, and Conchos. Marín listed these tribes as living in the La Junta vicinity in 1693 (Hackett 1926:391–95). In 1684 a Conchos head chief declared he had been for some 42 years the governor of a group of nations including Obomes (Oposmes), Polacmes, Posalmes, Cacalotitos, Mesquites, Conejos, Julimes, and Conchos (Sauer 1934:64). From 1688 to 1694, however, a Julimes Indian, Don Nicolás, was the governor of most if not all of the La Junta tribes, as well as the Julimes of San Antonio de Julimes above Cuchillo Parado. The many references to the La Junta tribes at this period give us little information regarding their culture, other than that the Patarabueyes were coming in close contact with Spanish culture, that they had trade and friendly relations with the Cibolas and Jumanos, and that they were usually at war with the more nomadic Indians surrounding them, including the Chisos, Sumas, and Apaches.

9

The Patarabueyes
1695–1800(?)

In 1712 or 1713 some Indians from La Junta had visited Colonel Don Juan Joseph Masoni at San Francisco de Cuellar and asked him to send missionaries to La Junta. As a result he sent Fray Andrés Ramirez to the La Junta pueblos, "where he had been on previous occasions." As a result of Ramirez's reply in 1713, the Trasviña Retís expedition was ordered. The following data are abstracted from the Trasviña Retís diary and accompanying papers, as translated by Reindorp (1938).

In 1715 Don Juan Antonio de Trasviña Retís, of San Francisco de Cuellar, accompanied by the Franciscans Fray Joseph de Arrangegui, Fray Gregorio Osorio, Fray Juan Antonio García, 30 soldiers, and numerous Indians, journeyed to La Junta to make a survey and census of the Patarabueyes and to reestablish the missions there.

Immediately above Cuchillo Parado on the Rio Conchos the Spaniards found the Chalome pueblo of San Pedro and a short distance beyond it the pueblo of Nuestra Señora de Begoña "where Indians of the eight pueblos of La Junta live." There were 28 Indians in this rancheria. They cultivated wheat and other grain and had a church. Only a few of the houses in the pueblo "had doors like a presidio."

A short distance below Cuchillo Parado they came to the pueblo of El Mesquite, which was renamed Nuestra Señora de Loreto. This pueblo had a central plaza and a defensive wall. Its houses and "portals" had thin walls and roof-beams of sycamore. There were 80 Indians in this pueblo, which was situated in the open valley land of the Rio Conchos, surrounded by irrigated fields of wheat, corn, and legumes.

One league farther down the Rio Conchos the expedition came to the pueblo of San Juan Bautista of the Cacalote nation, with 165 inhabitants.

This pueblo also had a defensive wall, and a plaza which the houses faced, and in which they met the Spaniards. Here also were fields of wheat, corn, and other grains.

Four leagues downstream at the juction of the Rio Conchos and the Rio Grande they came to the pueblo of San Francisco de la Junta (see Map) of the Oposme nation, the center of the eight La Junta pueblos. Here the Spaniards were met by Indians from all the pueblos with their governors, and captains, carrying flags of peace, and drawn up in orderly lines along the entrance to the pueblo. This pueblo was separated into three divisions about three hundred yards apart, and had 180 inhabitants. The governor of the pueblo of San Antonio de Julimes, named Don Juan Antonio de la Cruz, was a native of this pueblo.

One and one-half leagues up the Rio Grande from San Francisco was the pueblo of Nuestra Señora de Aranzazu of the Conejo nation, inhabited by 71 persons. Across the Rio Grande and below the junction (see Map) was the largest of the pueblos, Nuestra Señora de Guadalupe* of the Polacme and Cibola nations, two groups united for mutual defense against the nomadic Indians, who had attacked them on several occasions. This pueblo was well built and had two plazas; it was occupied by 550 Indians. Below this town, on both banks of the joined rivers, were three pueblos: Señor San José of the Pulique nation with 92 persons; San Antonio de Padua of the Conchos nation with 87 occupants; and San Cristóbal† of the Poxalma nation with 180 inhabitants (see Map). Altogether, and excepting the Conejo Indians of Nuestra Señora de Begoña of Cuchillo Parado, there were 1405 Indians in the La Junta pueblos and rancherias. The 190 Cholome Indians of San Pedro pueblo above Cuchillo Parado were not included in this count.

The effects of long contact with the Spaniards were by now quite apparent in the La Junta pueblos. Trasviña Retís was

> pleased to see Indians with such good reason and so polite without having had any education and also to see them so well-dressed, men as well as women, the chiefs and their wives being outstanding with better clothes in the Spanish fashion, with shirts of fine white linen worked in silk. Some had skirts of serge, silk shawls, Cordoba shoes and imported Brussels silk socks. I found men, women and children with good-natured, happy faces, who were very sociable with the Spaniards as they came and went all day long in the house where I was stopping; coming and going like servants with no differences and without showing the slightest action contrary to good loyalty.

There were already churches in several of the pueblos, and the fields were irrigated, a custom not previously noted. The Indians asked the Spaniards for an iron bar to use in opening ditches, and for plowshares, pickaxes, and

---

*Guadalupe is now placed at the present site of Ojinaga, Chihuahua. See Preface–1986. (J.C.K.)
†Now placed at the location given above for Guadalupe. (J.C.K.)

hoes, as well as for bells and adornments for their churches. Trasviña Retís notes: "In order to buy clothes, they travel more than one hundred leagues at the risk of meeting enemies to work on the farm estates of San Bartolomé Valley." At the time of his visit, 80 La Junta Indians were away working in the San Bartolomé fields, a practice which he attempted to halt.

On the way back to San Francisco de Cuellar, Trasviña Retís sent sheep and goats back to La Junta for the use of the priests.[1] The Patarabueyes at this time had close relationships with certain Apaches, who may have been Jumanos (see Chapter 6), but were confirmed enemies of the Chisos and other nomadic Indians of the region. They professed little knowledge of the country at any great distance from La Junta, except for the Conchos valley, and to a lesser extent the Rio Grande valley above and below La Junta for some distance. Trasviña Retís recommended that permanent missions be established at La Junta but that no Spanish settlers be sent there. He also asked that several hundred head of cattle and sheep be sent to the people there.

Acting on this recommendation, the Duke of Linares dispatched six priests to La Junta in 1716, and the missions of Nuestro Señor la Redonda del Collame, Nuestro Señor Padre San Francisco, San Pedro del Cuchillo Parado, San Juan, and San Cristóbal were founded. It was noted at this time that "the said Indians . . . are . . . very clever and politic, . . . those of the Cumano and Zíbola nations being especially well disposed" (Hackett 1937:408).[2]

The new missions were supplied with cows, sheep, and "tools for the cultivation of the land." Two years passed "with great spiritual and temporal increase." The supervision of the churches, and the care of the church cattle were left to Francisco, the Indian governor, who was a devout Christian and a regular seasonal worker in the fields of San Bartolomé.

The cattle led to the downfall of the missions. Some of them strayed to the country of the non-Christian Indians beyond the Rio Conchos, where the priests could not go. Francisco demanded their return, but the hostile Indians refused. Angered by this event, they conspired to kill the priests, who heard of it and fled, accompanied by Francisco. The priests barely escaped being ambushed, but reached Collame (the modern town of Coyame) safely, and eventually arrived in Chihuahua.

There they asked the Marquis of Valero to establish a presidio at La Junta and to send Spanish settlers there, but this request was refused. The priests then returned to La Junta and remained there, apparently without incident, until 1725. In that year there occurred an Indian uprising and the two youths who helped the missionaries were killed, while the missionaries were tied up, ready for execution. News of the revolt had reached Chihuahua, however, and a relief expedition reached La Junta in time to rescue the priests.

Presumably the La Junta missions were not again opened until sometime in 1732 or 1733, although there is some evidence to the contrary.[3] Menchero noted that in 1731 the Indian generals, governors, and other officials of the La Junta missions appeared in Chihuahua and begged him to send missionaries to reopen their churches. He accordingly requested the governor of Chihuahua to escort two priests to La Junta, and later, this being refused, he asked that the governor allow the priests to go alone. Six months later this had not been done, so Menchero sent other priests to La Junta, where they still were in 1744, one (Father Francisco Bravo Larchundia) "having founded three pueblos of Indians whom he instructed and reduced."

Menchero again asked for the establishment of a presidio at La Junta, noting the richness of the mines and fields there, and arguing that such a fortress would halt the depredation of the hostile Indians, "for the place is a passage and exit for many nations of Zibolas and Apaches." The presidio was not established for many years, but apparently from this time on, the missions were maintained constantly at La Junta. The Father Provincial noted in 1750 that after 1725, "at times two religious have resided in these missions, at others three, and sometimes four." He added that, "The said missions are exposed to constant attacks and hostilities of the enemy without recourse to a presidio nearby or to any other safeguard to their lives," and that "even when six or fewer religious were there no stipend whatever was given by the *real hacienda*."[4]

During this interval several expeditions visited La Junta, including those of Idoiaga and Vidaurre in 1747 and Rabago y Teran in 1748.[5] I have not seen the documents relative to these expeditions. Sauer notes that Idoiaga "took *padrones,* among others of the Cholome and Cíbolo tribes, the latter the 'Sibolos de San Xtobal, Puliques, y Pescados.'" The Cibolas were still well represented in the Rio Grande settlements.

In 1753 the Conde de Revilla-Gigedo visited La Junta in order to place missionaries there. At that time the list of missions included San Francisco, San Cristóbal (of the Cocoimes), and San Pedro (Revilla-Gigedo 1753, original manuscript). In the same year the Conde de Revilla-Gigedo noted that the congregation of the mission of San Francisco de Bizarron in Coahuila had been considerably enlarged by the presence of numerous "julimes venados, cibolos nortenos y cholomes" who were fugitives from Nueva Vizcaya, and who were hostile, "degenerate," and suspected of acting as spies for the Lipan (Portillo 1886:312–23).[6] In 1794 Father Trigo wrote, "I have not discussed the six missions at La Junta de los Ríos because I have not visited them. I know that they are fifty leagues east of the villa of Chihuahua, and I am told that their Indians are good, and that because they have no lands to sow they make frequent visits to Chihuahua, where they acquire by labor what is necessary for their maintenance; they are very keen in looking for work, and not at all lazy" (Hackett 1937:468). In 1759 Don Narciso Tapia reportedly visited La Junta, but I have no notes regarding his account (Tapia 1759, original manuscript).

Apparently, the La Junta missions were at times temporarily abandoned by the Spaniards during this period, for Father Lezaún noted that his missionary expedition there in 1759(?) was the third such *entrada* he had made (Hackett 1937:498). The question of establishing a presidio at La Junta had been raised again by the Conde de Revilla-Gigedo in 1752, but no action was taken until 1760. At that time Lezaún wrote:

> Our entrance (this was the third) was accomplished by promising the Indians that the presidio should be placed at a distance of ten leagues from the settlement [the pueblo of Nuestra Señora de Guadalupe de La Junta], as is ordered by the señor viceroy, so that they should not suffer damage to their fields and pueblos; but all has failed, and the promise has not been kept nor has the presidio been placed where it was ordered. It is being constructed at a distance of three squares [*quadras*] from the mission of Guadalupe, whereby the Indians are much disturbed; and not the least cause of their exasperation is the damage that their crops and their sheep, cattle, mules and horses suffer at the hands of the captain and soldiers of the presidio. From all this it is expected that those [Indians] who have remained will take flight, as other pueblos have done, and as a part of that of Guadalupe and the other two are now doing. [Lezaún, in Hackett 1937:499]

At this time there were six different missions and five missionaries at La Junta, but so serious was the political situation that the pueblos were speedily being abandoned. In 1761 the pueblo of San Juan at La Junta had lost half of its population of four hundred, and it was feared that an equal percentage of the total La Junta population of 2,350 Indians had fled (Hackett 1937:500).[7] Serrano attributed the abandonment of the La Junta pueblos, which were in a "state of discredit, ruin, and decadence," not only to a "desire to be free to confederate with the heathen nations and attack the kingdom, but also because these Indians are attempting to evade the tyrannies with which the [political and military officials] oppress them." He complained bitterly that the Indians were

> indulged in their vices, dances, *estufas*, superstitions, witchcrafts, and idolatries in the mountains, while we [the priests] receive no favor, but on the contrary are interfered with when we try to compel the vicious and rebellious to receive their instruction and catechism. On the one hand they give them protection in their disobedience to us, and on the other they harass and oppress them... [Serrano, in Hackett 1937:492]

The troublesome state of affairs at La Junta seems to have continued, since the presidio of Belén, established only in 1760, was moved to Julimes pueblo in 1766 (Bancroft 1886, 1889:585; Bancroft does not give the source of this statement). The fate of the La Junta Indians after this date is not given in any documentary source to which I have had access. In 1778 Escalante wrote that he preached at La Junta to the three Indian nations that were established there: the Conchos, the Julimes, and the Chocolomes (Bandelier 1890:85n.).[8] I have no further reference to La Junta prior to 1851, at which date an Anglo-American settlement was established there (Casey 1933:10–15). Documentary material of Anglo-American origin after this date contains notes regarding Apache and Comanche Indians in the La Junta vicinity, but there is no mention of the La Junta tribes in any of the sources to which I have had access. It is probable that most of the La Junta peoples, who had become increasingly acculturated by Spanish contact, were slowly absorbed into the rising tide of Spanish settlement. Today San Francisco de La Junta and Pulicos are Mexican towns situated on the sites of the ancient Indian pueblos of the same name, and there is no indication that these towns were ever abandoned.[9] Already in 1760 Spanish settlement of the Conchos valley was well underway, and must have reached La Junta by 1800, if not before (Lezaún, in Hackett 1937:478).[10]

In June, 1937, I made enquiries in the La Junta vicinity and found, surprisingly perhaps, that all tradition of the Patarabueyes, or related groups, had not been completely lost. Several informants remembered the "Trigos" and Cholome Indians. These, some said, had drifted southward into Mexico when the Apaches came. The other La Junta Indians who lived in the old towns had finally been gathered into the one pueblo of Pulicos by the priests, in order that they might be administered to more easily. There they had become totally acculturated.

One informant, Jesús Alvarez, of Presidio, Texas, had heard stories from the older people about the "civilized" Indians who once lived there. The "Cholombos" Indians, according to his story, were still living near La Junta when the Anglo-American occupation began, and the American and Mexican army forces killed off the last of these Indians.[11] He also recalled the Conchos, Mansos, and Julimeno Indians without prompting, but the older names for the Patarabueyes were unfamiliar to him.

Several of the more elderly "Mexican" occupants of the La Junta valley claimed descent from the old, settled tribes there, proudly differentiating their "civilized" Indian ancestry from the "savage" Apache ancestry of other local citizens. Thus, in all probability, is explained the final disappearance of the sedentary Indians of La Junta.

The Patarabueyes, ca. 1535–1800
Summary

The history of the Patarabueye Indians at La Junta de los Rios has been traced in detail from 1535(?) or 1582, until their disappearance as an ethnic entity about 1800. There are only two gaps of significance in that historical record. The "People of the Cows" of de Vaca cannot be identified for certain as the Patarabueyes of the 1580s. Secondly, there is a gap between the Patarabueyes of the 1580s and the La Junta tribes of Conchos affiliation from 1680 onward. The latter apparent gap in all probability can be explained merely as a change in nomenclature applied to the La Junta tribes, since the same pueblos were occupied in the two periods, and the culture of the Patarabueyes of 1582–83 appears identical with that of the La Junta groups of 1683 and 1715. However, the change in tribal nomenclature[12] is so great and so relatively abrupt that further evidence must be adduced. Fortunately there is conclusive archaeological evidence of the continuity in occupation and in culture of the prehistoric and historic La Junta pueblos. These archaeological data are presented in Part IV, together with comparative archaeological data for the Jumanos.

The detailed history of the Patarabueye Indians from 1535(?) to about 1800, terminating in their acculturation and absorption into the Mexican ethnic melting pot, stands in striking contrast to the history of the Jumano Indians from 1583 to 1771, which terminated in the absorption of that group into the great Apache stock. The contrast between Jumano and Patarabueye cultures is likewise striking; this contrast is emphasized further by the archaeological data presented in the following pages.

Part IV

Archaeological Data: Patarabueyes and Jumanos

10
Patarabueye Archaeology

Fortunately, it is unnecessary to depend solely upon the documentary sources for our knowledge of the Jumanos and Patarabueyes. The archaeological sites of many of the historic Patarabueye villages have been identified and two of them have been partially excavated. Excavations have been made in one prehistoric Patarabueye site and surface collections are available from many related sites, both prehistoric and historic. Patarabueye archaeology is therefore comparatively well known. The archaeology of the Jumano Indians is less well known; no archaeological sites that definitely can be identified as Jumano camps have been located. Nevertheless, such archaeological data as we have aid considerably in elucidating the Jumano problem. There emerges a general picture of two distinct archaeological cultures sharing many basic traits and having some detailed items in common.

The documentary sources have provided certain criteria that must be used in identifying the archaeological remnants of Patarabueye culture. Sites identified as Patarabueye must be localized geographically in the general region of La Junta and must show long continued occupancy. The sites must be those of an agricultural people who dwelled in permanent villages of large houses and pithouses and utilized the bow and arrow. These sites must be distinctive for the region, must show associated European trade objects, and finally must be identifiable, at least in part, with the locations of specific pueblos described in the documentary sources.

All of these criteria are present in the archaeological culture which has been named the Bravo Valley Aspect, particularly in the Concepción and Conchos foci of this aspect (Kelley 1939:221–24). E. B. Sayles first recognized and described this archaeological culture, using the term "Jumano Phase" for those components situated on the Texas side of the Rio Grande (Sayles 1935:79–84, Plate 12, Map E, Tables 7, 9, 13), and "Conchos Phase" for the corresponding components on the Chihuahua side (Sayles 1936:84, 107).[1] Sites of the Bravo Valley Aspect are distributed along the Rio Grande from the vicinity of Redford, Texas, to a point far upstream from the mouth of the Rio Conchos, and along most of the lower course of the latter stream (Fig. 10). The Conchos Focus, as used here, includes components belonging principally to the fully historic or mission period, presumably dating from about 1700 onward. The Concepción Focus includes components of both the later prehistoric and the early historic periods, and represents the culture of the Patarabueyes as described in the reports of the Rodríguez and Espejo *entradas.* An earlier and completely prehistoric phase of this occupation, the La Junta Focus, has likewise been identified.

The La Junta Focus

This focus is best illustrated at the Millington site (Shafter 7:1), situated just east of Presidio, Texas, on the low terrace of the Rio Grande adjoining a former channel of that stream. For several hundred yards along the terrace edge, scattered fire-cracked stones, animal bone fragments, flint chips, and artifacts indicate the former presence of an extensive village. Toward the center of the area there is a broad but low midden, black with charcoal. At the eastern end of this midden, refuse heaps rise several feet above the present surface. This site has been identified as the Santiago pueblo of the Espejo expedition, and as the pueblo of Nuestra Señora de Guadalupe de La Junta of the eighteenth century historians.* In the initial stratigraphic test made at this site in 1936 it was noted that approximately the lower half of the midden debris contained no artifacts of Spanish origin, although these appeared in profusion in the upper few inches of the deposits, but was, instead, characterized by sherds of El Paso Polychrome and other Southwestern pottery types largely of Chihuahua culture affiliation. This ceramic complex was later found at other sites and locally is diagnostic of the La Junta Focus (Plate II*j-n,* and possibly *r-t*).

Later excavations at the Millington site revealed that many pithouses and one near-surficial "pueblo" structure contained similar pottery. Rectangular houses, averaging about 11 by 14 feet, built in shallow or deep pits were the oldest type of dwelling found. These houses usually possessed adobe floors, and occasionally had low adobe curbs surrounding the floor (Plate I*C*). They were oriented north and south and were occasionally built

---

*See Preface–1986 for a correction of this identification. (J.C.K.)

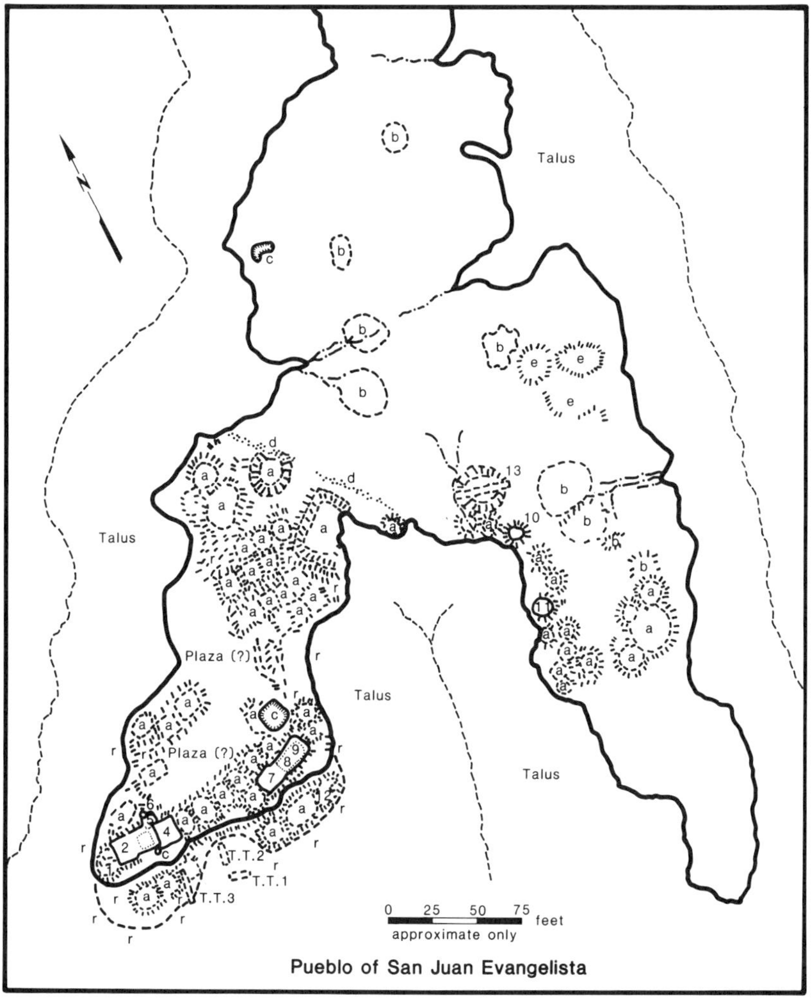

Figure 3. The Loma Alta site (Shafter 7:3).

side by side to form east-west tiers of rooms. Vertical walls of jacale construction were built independently of the pit walls. Roof supports were either placed at the corners of the rooms or were set into the room a few feet from the corners. Entrance was presumably through the roof since no trace of side entrances could be found, and the roofs were probably flat, or nearly so. In most of the La Junta Focus houses of this type, a rectangular block of plastered adobe had been set on the floor adjoining the center of the south wall. Shallow adobe-lined fire basins were frequently found immediately to

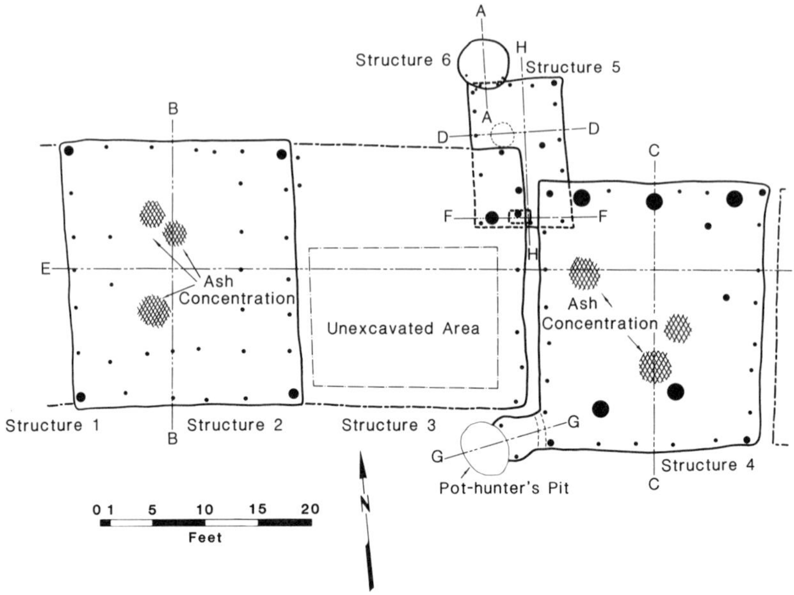

Figure 4. House group I, Loma Alta site.

the north of these altar-like structures. Many irregular pits cut into the house floors or into midden debris were noted; these usually contained refuse but were occasionally used for inhumation of the dead. In addition to the rectangular adobe pithouses, several small unlined circular or oval house pits were assigned to this focus. These pits had pole superstructures, but no other structural details are known. They may represent storage houses, or perhaps they were the temporary dwellings of visiting hunters.

Artifacts of the La Junta Focus, aside from pottery, include small triangular, side-notched, or tanged arrowpoints, small flake sidescrapers or knives, double-pointed beveled knives, small flake drills or awls, snub-nosed flake scrapers, crude chipped handaxes (Plate III), shaped rectangular and unshaped one-hand manos, shallow oval-bowl metates, carved stone bowls, transverse grooved arrow-shaft straighteners of polished stone (notable for their pointed extension handles or hafting tangs), tubular stone "cloud-blower" type pipes, and numerous small flattish ovate pebbles notched at both ends (Plate IV). Many artifacts of shell and bone likewise were found, including long tubular beads of bird leg bone, *Olivella* and *Conus* shell beads, shell discs, and "spoon-shaped" artifacts of conch shell (Plate III). Aside from pottery, little difference can be detected between the artifacts of the La Junta Focus and those of the subsequent Concepción Focus.

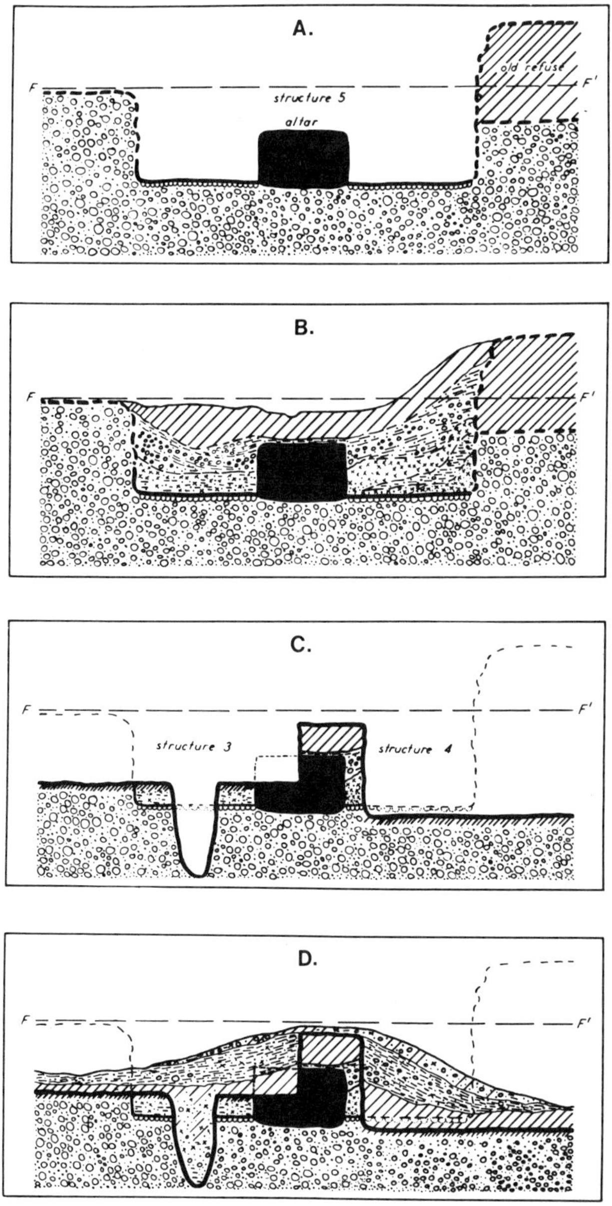

Figure 5. Sequence of events at the Loma Alta site. *A*. Structure 5, La Junta Focus, cut into gravel and old refuse of unknown provenance. *B*. Structure 5 abandoned and refilled with fallen roof debris, gravel, and fine sediment, and at the top by a layer of refuse. *C*. Structures 3 and 4, Concepción Focus, cut into fill of Structure 5, destroying part of walls, floor, and altar of Structure 5. *D*. Structures 3 and 4 abandoned and refilled with washed gravel, silts, and sand mixed with older refuse.

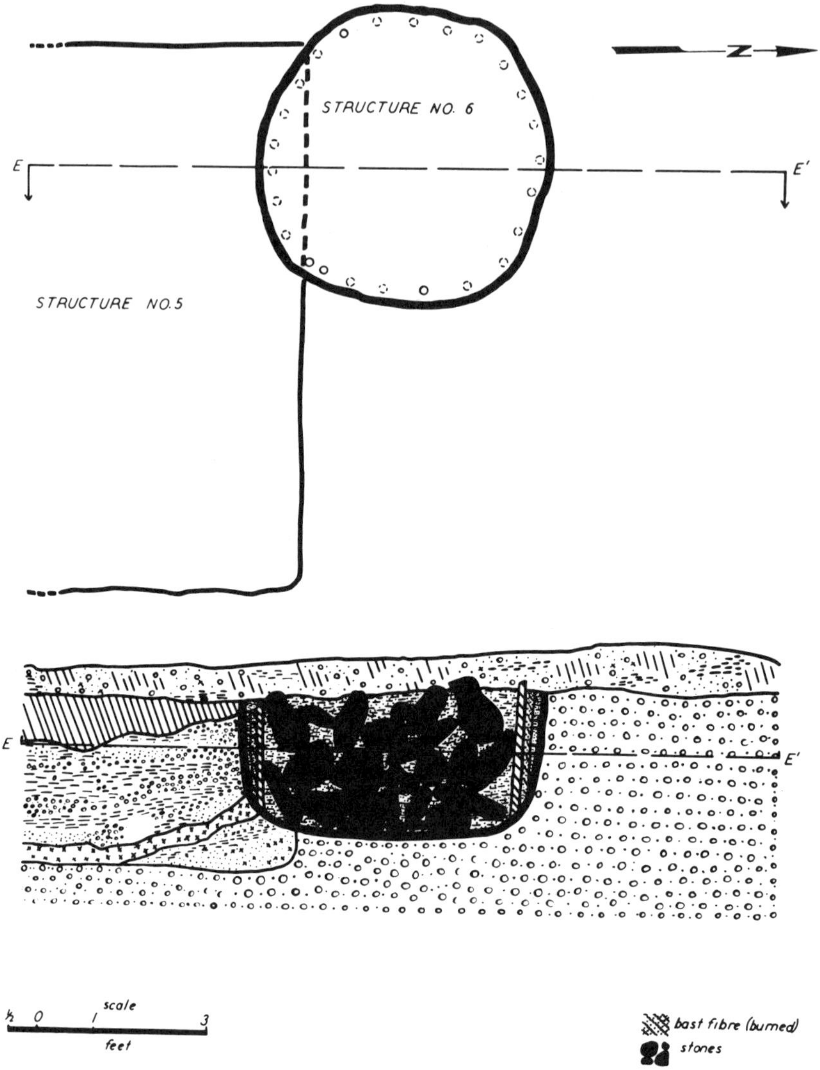

Figure 6. The Loma Alta site (Shafter 7:3). Structure 6 intersecting Structure 5.

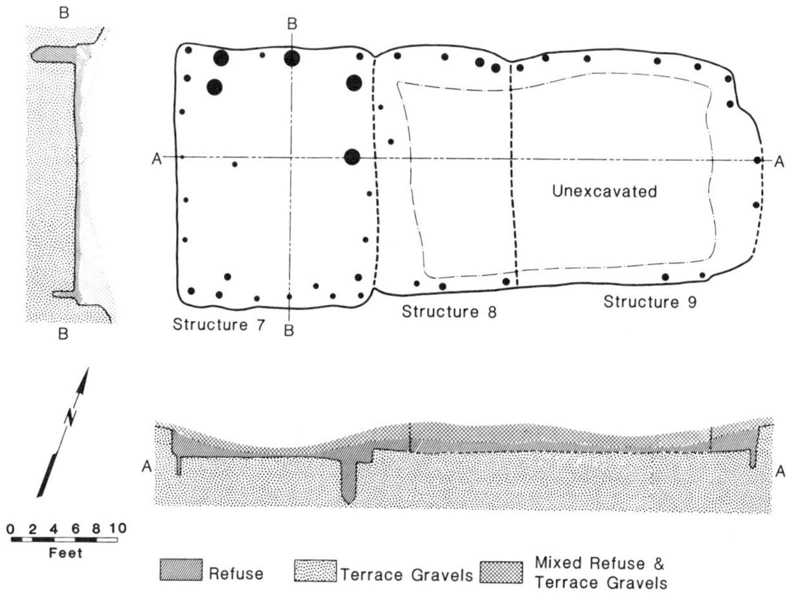

Figure 7. House group II, the Loma Alta site.

La Junta Focus houses have been excavated also at the Shiner site (Shafter 6:1), the late occupation of which appears to belong entirely to this focus, and at the Loma Alta site (Shafter 7:3; see Fig. 4, structure 6). This focus seems to be present in almost all Bravo Valley sites; in all such sites it is the oldest horizon (Figs. 5, 9), and the one during which the thickest layers of midden debris accumulated. On the basis of the associated Southwestern pottery types of fairly well-known age, the La Junta Focus is assigned to the period ca. A.D. 1200–1400.

The Concepción Focus

In the original Millington site stratigraphic test, the strata overlying the La Junta debris and underlying the surficial layers rich in European artifacts contained plain brown, reddish, gray, or red-on-gray pottery of previously unknown types. Some of the vessels represented appeared to be somewhat conical in form with pointed or rounded bottoms, cylindrical

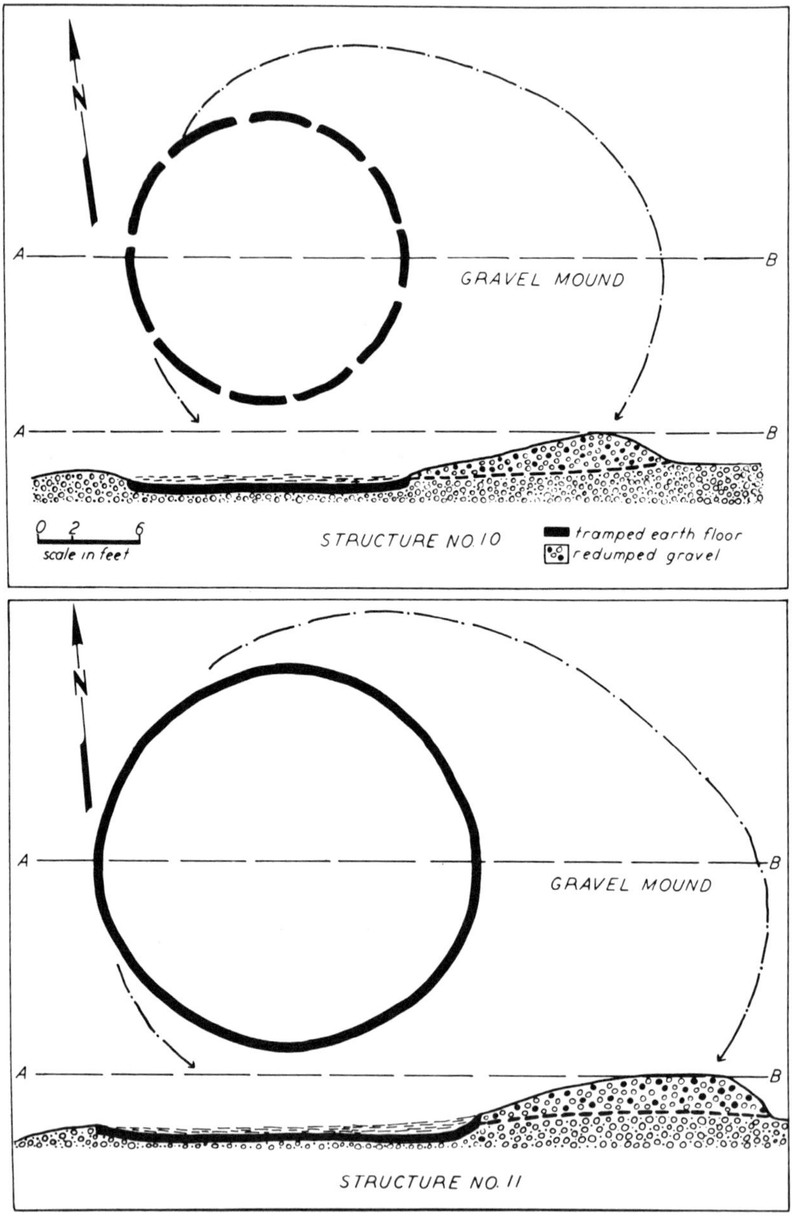

Figure 8. Structures 10, 11, the Loma Alta site.

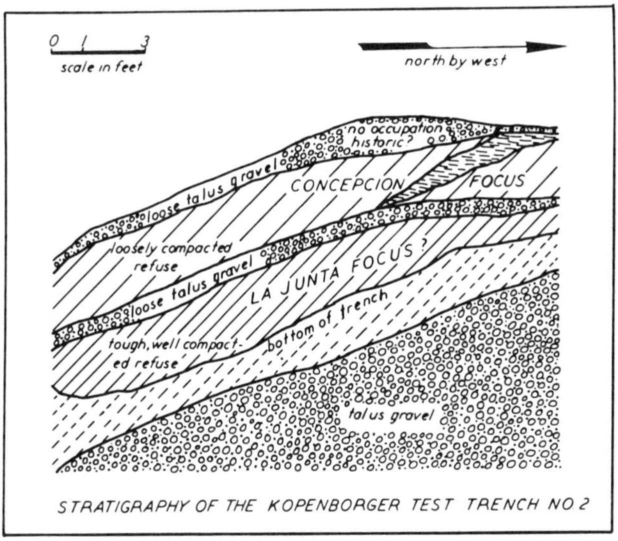

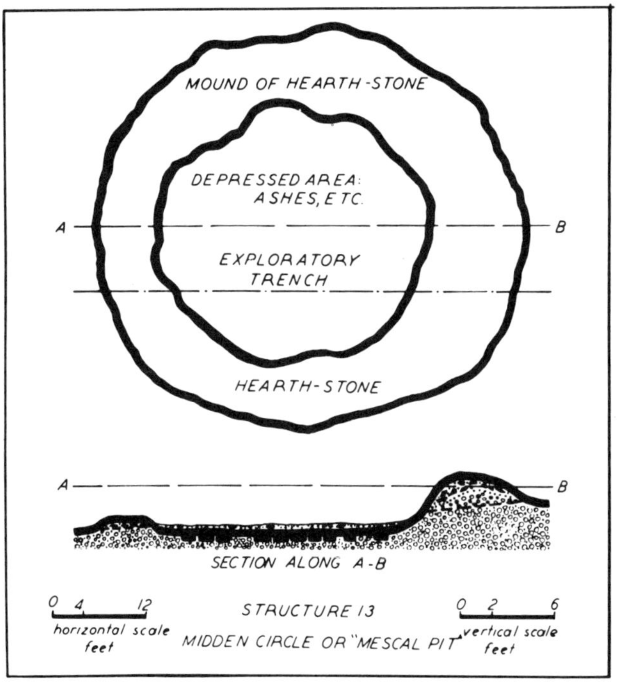

Figure 9. Structure 13 and stratigraphy, the Loma Alta site.

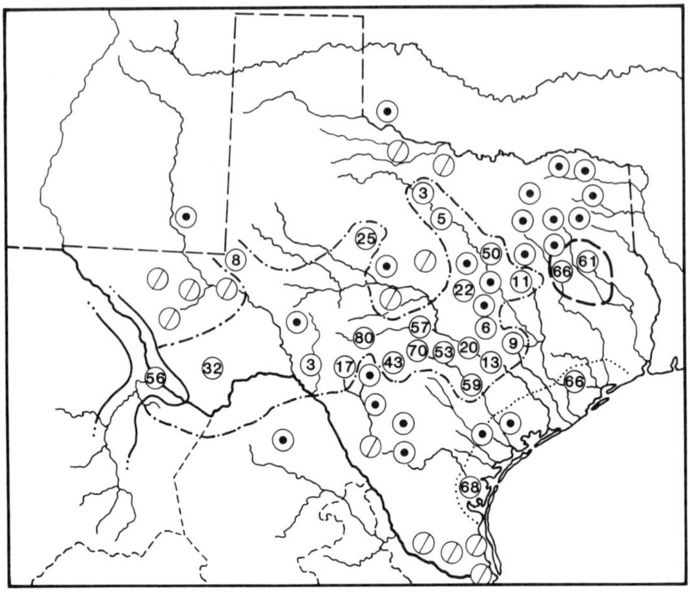

·—·—Toyah Focus —— Bravo Valley Aspect — — Allen and Frankston foci

·······Rockport and Galveston foci ㉕ Percentage of Perdiz Pointed Stem in collection

⊙ Less than one percent Perdiz ⊘ No Perdiz in collection

Figure 10. Distribution of Perdiz Pointed Stem and the Toyah Focus.

necks, and slightly outflaring rims. Plain, neck-banded, and vertically striated varieties of this ware have been noted (Plate II*a-c*). It was later discovered that similar pottery wares were associated with houses of a type somewhat different from those of the La Junta Focus. This combination of pottery types and house types was termed the Concepción Focus. The Concepción Focus was best represented at the Loma Alta site, which has therefore been named the type site of the focus, although similar houses and pottery were found at the Millington site.

The Loma Alta site (Shafter 7:3) is situated on the top of a high mesa or second terrace of the Rio Grande some five miles west of Presidio and directly opposite the mouth of the Rio Conchos, the original "La Junta" (see Map). In this vicinity the high terrace is a long narrow tongue-like extension of the main high terrace mass. This extension splits into two wings near the edge of the valley. On the surface of the western wing the depressions of several tiers of pithouses with associated areas of midden debris and level plaza enclosures were visible (Fig. 3). Other house pits could be seen at the contact of the talus slope with the southern tip of the mesa, on a somewhat lower level than the mesa top houses, and the talus slope itself, especially on the south, was littered with midden debris. At the north the remains of a stone wall serve to isolate the western mesa, although there is no assurance that the wall is of the same age as the village. On the adjoining eastern wing of the mesa there was a ring-midden of fire-cracked stone (Fig. 9) and along its western edge, facing the village ruin across the canyon, the floors of circular lodges, surrounded by banked-up mesa gravels and fire-cracked stones, were found. It has been suggested that the lodges were either the remains of a temporary encampment of some nomadic group, such as the Jumanos, or else the sweat houses or storage houses of the main village. On the low terrace below the high mesa and adjoining the old river channel, another ruin, attributed to the Concepción Focus, was discovered. This is perhaps the group of flat-roofed houses forming a sort of "suburb" to the village noted by Luxán.

Several of the Concepción Focus houses at the Loma Alta site were excavated wholly or in part and the type is well known. The houses were large, averaging 24 by 28 feet, and were customarily placed side by side to form long east-west tiers. The individual houses were rectangular, almost square, constructed in individual pits ranging from a few inches to several feet in depth (Figs. 3, 4, 7). Vertical jacale walls, built just inside the pit, in association with a central superstructure supported by four or more large posts, often over a foot and a half in diameter, set in a rectangular arrangement several feet away from the walls, suggests the presence of a flat roof as described in historical accounts. The floors were of hard-packed refuse and earth; no adobe curbs or altars were found, nor was there any trace of a side entrance. One house (Fig. 4, structure 4), however, possessed a curious circular appendage at the southwest corner, representing either an attached storage room or possibly an entrance anteroom. One somewhat similar circular subterranean storage room was found a few feet to the north of the same house group (Figs. 4, 6). On the floor of each house there were two, three, or even more, accumulations of white ash suggesting the contemporaneous usage of several floor hearths. This, taken together with the large size of the structures, suggests that each housed several hearth groups, possibly representing an extended family.

Each house had been constructed separately, and in one house group (Fig. 4) the pits varied in depth from house to house. In the same house group one house had obviously been constructed as a sort of lean-to structure utilizing the house walls of the adjoining structures. Even though constructed separately, the houses were placed in planned rows. Although they sometimes diverged slightly from the row, owing to minor differences in house lengths or placement, it is apparent that each row in the final stage of development represented one long continuous dwelling. Such buildings were obviously those described by the historians, and in somewhat smaller form are still built locally by the modern descendants of the ancients (Plate I*A*), although the gabled roof of the modern structures is probably of Spanish introduction.

There was a notable difference in size between the houses of the La Junta and Concepción foci, and the difference was emphasized by the lack of adobe floors, curbs, altars, and fire pits in the Concepción Focus houses. Furthermore, the changes in house type seem to indicate a change in social custom as well. The houses of the two foci had in common their rectangular shape, north-south orientation of individual houses, placements of houses in east-west tiers, construction of houses in pits, jacale walls, central superstructure, and, presumably, flat roofs and roof entrances. Houses transitional in type were excavated at the Millington site. These structures indicate that the Concepción-type houses may have developed from large, somewhat open shelters attached to the northern ends of the La Junta-type houses. The evidence in the same transitional examples is that the La Junta houses with their altars may have at the same time been relegated to the role of isolated ceremonial structures.

Large circular pithouses or earth-lodge structures resembling Pawnee lodges in ground plan also were found at the Millington site (see Kelley 1939 for a description). These houses appear to belong to the Concepción Focus, although their stratigraphic position is not certain. One such circular house was definitely later than La Junta Focus houses, which had been partially destroyed during its construction. This structure contained an adobe altar of the type common in rectangular houses of the La Junta Focus. These circular houses apparently had flat roofs and roof entrances, although the evidence in this regard is not completely convincing. They may be regarded as the flat-roofed pithouses built in the fields, described by historians, or alternatively they may represent the habitations of some group such as the Jumanos.

Artifacts of stone, bone, and shell of the Concepción Focus appear to be very similar, if not identical, in type with those of the preceding La Junta Focus. Deep circular mortar holes in large igneous boulders may perhaps be new. In pottery, however, there is an absolute break with the previous period. Gone are the intrusive wares from New Mexico and northern Chihuahua. In their place is the interesting assemblage of plain wares already noted in association with rare red-on-gray or red-on-brown wares. The common household ware seems to be Chinati Plain (Plate II*a*) or the associated variants, Chinati Striated-Neck and Chinati Neck-Banded (Plate II*b, c*). Chinati ware is a somewhat sandy ware with gray, brown, or reddish-brown paste. The principal shape is that shown in Plate II*a* but many examples have a true pointed bottom, giving a Woodland-like appearance to the jars. Hemispherical bowls are also known from the

Millington site collections but these may not have appeared until late in the period. In addition to the neck-striated and neck-banded varieties shown, there are rare examples with a row of punctate marks around the neck. The surface finish of the Chinati wares ranges from very rough to semi-polished. Apparently no slip was applied. The general appearance and range of shapes and surface texturing in Chinati is suggestive of Alma Plain and the associated textured wares of the Mogollon culture to the northwest (Haury 1936:32–40). Similarities with plain wares found along the Texas coast are likewise apparent.

In addition to Chinati ware, many sherds of an unnamed polished or semi-polished red ware, often slipped or washed, were found in the Concepción Focus houses at the Loma Alta site (Plate II*c*). In form this ware seems to have varied from the Chinati-type shape to a more globular-bodied olla with shorter neck. This ware also appeared in the form of straight-rimmed semi-hemispherical bowls. This was a sand-tempered ware with a moderately fine paste, usually brownish or reddish in color. The exterior was well smoothed and often polished over the thin red slip or wash. Smoothing of the surface produced a curious rippled effect in some instances. Here again, the resemblance to wares of the Mogollon series is rather startling.

A few sherds of a red-on-gray (Paloma Red-on-Gray, Plate II*f*) and a red-on-brown ware (Capote Red-on-Brown, Plate II*g*) were found. At the Millington site, sherds of Paloma Red-on-Gray reveal the vessel form to be that of a small bowl or saucer with rounded or flattened bottom and vessel walls beveled out at the rim to form a broad flat lip painted with a red band. The interior design in red forms a near-floral pattern utilizing broad curving red lines on a thin gray wash. Capote Red-on-Brown has similar designs in red, crudely executed on unslipped brown paste. The rim in this ware is direct and unbeveled, and large hemispherical bowls, as well as rare ollas, are represented. This ware appears to have become extremely popular late in the Concepción Focus; in the following Conchos Focus, it developed into the cruder Conchos Red-on-Brown series (Plate II*h*).

Two trade sherds of great interest were found in the Concepción Focus debris at the Loma Alta site, one on a house floor, the other in the surficial midden debris. These sherds are unmistakably Patton Engraved (Plate II*u*; cf. Plate II*v*), the common pottery type of the early historic Allen Focus of the Neches River in eastern Texas (near present-day Beaumont). The Allen Focus has been identified by Krieger as the archaeological remnant of historic Hasinai or Tejas Indian culture (Krieger, personal communication). The presence of these sherds at Presidio, some 500 miles or more west of their place of origin, is striking confirmation of the reported trade relations maintained by the Jumanos at the dawn of the historic period between the Tejas and the Patarabueyes.

On the floor of one Loma Alta house of Concepción Focus affiliation, fragments of an iron knife or sword were found. This is the sole indication of historic contact at this site, although it was certainly visited by the Spaniards in 1582. The site was not again mentioned in the records, and pottery of European types so common in later sites of the Conchos Focus was not found there. The Loma Alta site, therefore, probably was abandoned between 1582 and the establishment of the La Junta missions in 1680. At the Millington site, debris of the La Junta Focus grades upward in the refuse heaps almost imperceptibly into that of the Concepción Focus and subsequently into that of the Conchos Focus. All the evidence points to continuous occupancy; at other sites the same situation is apparent wherever midden refuse has been exposed in cross-section. Only at the Loma Alta site does there appear to have been an earlier La Junta Focus settlement (Figs. 4, 5), followed by a later Concepción Focus occupation after an intervening period of abandonment. And since only a small portion of the latter site has been excavated, the evidence for discontinous occupancy is not overwhelming even there. In view of these circumstances the span of the Concepción Focus is estimated roughly at A.D. 1400–1700.

The Conchos Focus

In the upper few inches of midden debris at the Millington site, great quantities of thick red, red-on-brown, and red-on-cream pottery were found (Plate II*h*). Some of this pottery was wheel-turned; much of it was glazed wholly or in part in imitation of the Spanish style. Associated with this pottery complex and similar European wares were many items of metal (Plate III*D*), and bones of domesticated animals. One Spanish coin with a date in the 1750s was found. Such materials were especially numerous in the elevated refuse heaps at the eastern end of the site. They were likewise associated with certain late house structures similar in detail to the large single houses of the Concepción Focus, and with sparse remains of surface houses of unknown type. Again, alien-looking circular or oval structures, characterized in this instance by many close-set small support posts, possibly platform or floor supports, were found. Such stone objects as were found in debris of this period were similar to those of the Concepción Focus. The artifact complex represented must be referred, obviously, to the mission period of the eighteenth century, and serves to define the Conchos Focus.

Along the edge of the low terrace near the river lowlands a mile or so east of the Loma Alta village is an early Conchos Focus or terminal Concepción Focus site (Shafter 7:4) now badly reduced by erosion. No excavation was attempted at this site, and no consequent data were obtained on architectural features. The pottery, however, is of interest. Most of it is

Capote Red-on-Brown (Plate II*g*), and there is some Chinati Plain, Neck-Banded, and Striated-Neck (Plate II*a-c*). Majolica is very common (Plate II*o*), and one sherd collected here has been identified as Aztec ware in the late precolonial style[2] (Plate II*p*). Stone objects from the site are similar to those of the preceding periods. The site is obviously a late Concepción or very early Conchos Focus village (ca. A.D. 1680–1720) and illustrates the gradual transition into the mission period that occurred during the early eighteenth century.

Patarabueye Archaeology: Conclusions

The Concepción and Conchos foci sites and artifacts of the Presidio region are certainly those of the culture described in the historical records and attributed to the Patarabueye Indians. Continuous occupation of the area by the Patarabueyes from about A.D. 1200 until near the end of the eighteenth century, therefore, is indicated by the archaeological evidence. Cultural changes occurred during this time span, and the appearance of several new traits and the disappearance of former items around A.D. 1400 may indicate the entrance of foreign elements into the culture at that time. Nevertheless, evidence of any wide-spaced shift in population or any basic change in culture during these six centuries is completely lacking. Consequently, Sauer's theory that the Jumanos were in possession of the La Junta towns at the beginning of the historic period but were later driven out and replaced by Conchos Indians (Patarabueyes) expanding down the Rio Conchos is invalid, or else the assumption must be made that such slight difference in culture existed between Jumanos and Conchos that no archaeological evidence of the postulated change could be expected. In any event, the safest conclusion is that the culture participated in during the historic period by the Patarabueyes at La Junta was in itself an old established culture in this area and that in all probability the Patarabueyes themselves were likewise residents of long standing.

It is possible that the circular houses that appear as oddities at all periods of Bravo Valley Aspect history are to be attributed to some intrusive group such as the Jumanos, but on the basis of existing evidence such a conclusion seems unwarranted. Other elements in the culture likewise perhaps point eastward and northward: double-pointed beveled knives and snub-nosed scrapers are certainly of Plains origin, and Chinati ware itself looks Plains or Mogollon. However, these items seem to have been integral parts of the culture rather than intrusive traits. Only when we find such definite intrusives as the sherds of Patton Engraved ware are we sure of outside contacts. The Bravo Valley evidence, therefore, in itself tells us nothing regarding the archaeological remnants of Jumano culture. Jumano archaeology must be studied elsewhere in its own right.

11
Jumano Archaeology

Jumano history provides criteria for the identification of the archaeological remnants of Jumano culture. The general type of culture, the geographic range of the group, the time period represented, and known contacts with other groups are all classes of evidence that must be used. Furthermore, it seems improbable that the archaeological remains of such an important group as the Jumanos can have remained entirely unnoticed, even though many localities in Texas are not well known archaeologically. Identification of Jumano archaeological remains, then, would seem to be merely a matter of examining the known archaeological complexes with reference to the Jumano criteria. Unfortunately, this did not prove to be the case. Several archaeological foci have been isolated that conform to the criteria in varying degrees, none completely.

The following criteria were employed.

Culture

Jumano archaeological sites should represent the more or less transient camps of tipi-dwelling bison hunters. In view of the well-developed Jumano trade in bison hides, tools for the preparation of these hides should be included in the artifact lists. Presumably arrowpoints and associated implements should be included likewise. In terms of Texas archaeology, this means that Jumano sites should yield arrowpoints, snub-nosed scrapers, and specialized flint knives, probably of the double-pointed, beveled-edge variety so commonly used by the bison hunters of the Southern Plains.

Range

Sites of any archaeological complex identified as Jumano should occur in the following areas: (1) in the saline lake district of southeastern New Mexico and the southwestern Panhandle of Texas; (2) along the Pecos River and Toyah Creek, or alternatively Comanche Creek; (3) in the Trans-Pecos region, especially in the vicinity of La Junta; (4) along the modern-day Concho River (in Texas) and the middle drainage of the Colorado River; (5) along the southern and eastern fringes of the Edwards Plateau, principally near the headwaters of the Guadalupe River and similar streams; (6) perhaps, but not certainly so, in the region of the Anacacho Mountains and along the Rio Grande near Eagle Pass.

Chronology

Archaeological remains identified as Jumano should be referable to the late prehistoric and early historic periods. Such remains should, at least in part, be subject to chronological correlation with the Concepción Focus at La Junta and the Frankston and Allen foci in eastern Texas.

Contacts

In view of the intimate relations of the Jumanos with the Patarabueyes, Jumano archaeological remains should be recognizable to some degree in materials obtained from components of the Bravo Valley Aspect. Furthermore, it would seem probable, but not absolutely necessary, that Jumano artifacts should appear in Frankston Focus or Allen Focus components. Finally, some Jumano sites should yield artifacts of European origin.

Several archaeological complexes must be considered as possibly of Jumano origin. Among these are the Valley Creek Culture ("Wichita Phase"), the Henrietta Focus, the Nueces Focus, the Austin Focus, the Trading House Focus, the Toyah Focus, and the Livermore Focus. To this list must be added the Frankston and Allen foci and the Bravo Valley Aspect itself.

The Bravo Valley Aspect

Luxán noted that the Jumano Indians encountered on Toyah Creek in 1583 resembled the Patarabueyes in their style of clothing but not in their houses. If such scholars as Bolton and Sauer are correct in identifying Jumanos and Patarabueyes as one and the same people, this resemblance should go deeper than a similarity in clothing. Actually, in such an event, the Jumanos frequently found in western and central Texas would have to be regarded as bison-hunting Patarabueyes, and their archaeological culture accordingly should represent a stripped-down version of the Bravo Valley Aspect, lacking in permanent houses, agricultural equipment, and perhaps pottery and other items. All those traits of the Bravo Valley Aspect associated with the hunt, the types of projectile points, knives, scrapers, arrow-shaft tools, etc., logically should occur in the "Jumano" sites.

There is one bit of evidence, and the only one, that lends support to this hypothesis. In 1938 W. C. Holden excavated the Blue Mountain rockshelter in the caprock of the Southern Plains in Winkler County, Texas (Holden 1938:208–21). The culture revealed by this excavation is clearly identifiable with the Bravo Valley Aspect. In Holden's illustrations are visible all of the principal arrowpoint types of the Bravo Valley Aspect, and apparently in approximately the same numerical ratio in which they occur in the La Junta sites. Associated with these are plain and engraved tubes of bird bone characteristic of the Bravo Valley Aspect. Sherds of Chupadero Black-on-White also were found suggesting that either the La Junta Focus or the Concepción Focus of the aspect is represented.

Blue Mountain rockshelter is not far from that section of the Pecos River where the Jumanos were found in 1583, and is probably quite close to the locality in which they were visited by the Spaniards in the first decades of the seventeenth century. The principal associated pottery, Chupadero Black-on-White, is thought to have been in use from around A.D. 1300 to 1600, so that the site probably falls within the proper time horizon for such an identification.

This is convincing evidence and it seems conceivable, if not probable, that the Jumanos of this vicinity did have a Bravo Valley Aspect culture in the years between 1583 and 1623. But whatever the circumstances with regard to the early period, it seems certain that the later Jumanos of central and western Texas did not have a Bravo Valley Aspect culture, since the peculiar combination of projectile points characteristic of this group has not been found away from the La Junta region, except in the one instance of the Blue Mountain rockshelter.

The Frankston and Allen Foci

Sites of these foci, which have been identified, respectively, as the late prehistoric and early historic cultures of the Hasinai or Tejas Indians,[1] are found primarily in the Neches River valley in eastern Texas. In view of the fact that both foci represent sedentary agricultural groups whose known distribution only slightly overlaps the eastern periphery of the Jumano range (Figs. 10, 11), they both can safely be disregarded as possible Jumano cultures. Nevertheless, it is important to note that one of the common arrowpoint types of the Frankston Focus is Perdiz Stemmed, one of the diagnostic types of the Bravo Valley Aspect. Furthermore, as already

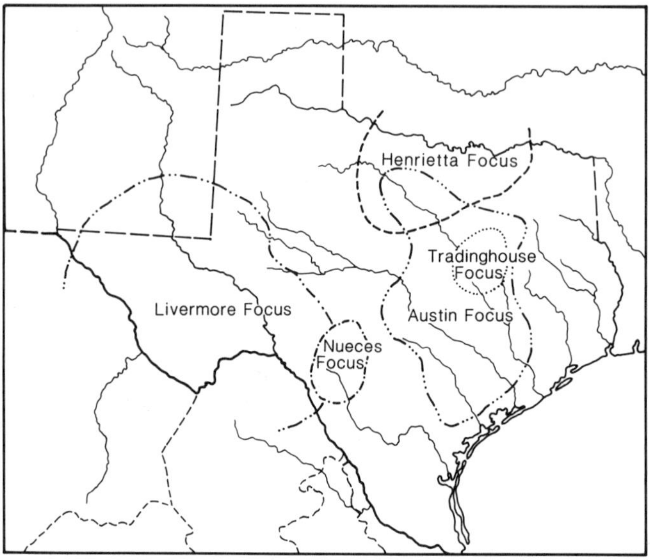

Figure 11. Distribution of late archaeological foci.

noted, two sherds of Patton Engraved pottery (Plate II*u, v*) of the Allen Focus were found in the Bravo Valley Aspcct site of Loma Alta, near La Junta. Primarily, such evidence serves to verify the recorded activity of the Jumanos as traders between the Patarabueyes and the Tejas, but, as will soon become apparent, an even greater significance can be inferred.

Valley Creek Culture ("Wichita Phase")

E. B. Sayles described an archaeological complex termed the "Wichita Phase" as the culture of a late hunting-agricultural group distributed over a broad zone stretching diagonally across Texas from northeast to southwest through the central part of the state (Sayles 1935). In the vicinity of Abilene, Texas, Cyrus N. Ray has described similar artifacts under the classificatory terms "Pottery Complex Artifacts" and "Small Scraper Culture" (Ray 1929, 1935). By mutual agreement, Ray's complexes were combined with Sayles's "Wichita Phase" and the resulting culture was renamed "Valley Creek Culture" (Ray and Sayles 1941:175–76). Valley Creek Culture covers much of the Jumano range and in other ways fulfills many of the requirements of a Jumano archaeological complex. However, the accumulation of new data by the Department of Anthropology of the University of Texas has made it necessary to split Valley Creek Culture into at least four archaeological foci: Henrietta, Austin, Nueces, and Toyah, each of which must be considered independently. The first three will be examined in this chapter; the Toyah Focus will be examined in the following chapter.

The Henrietta Focus

This focus represents the culture of unidentified late prehistoric bison hunters and farmers, and includes such artifacts as double-pointed beveled knives and snub-nosed scrapers (Krieger 1946:87–159). However, its range extended northward from Abilene through the Red River drainage, barely overlapping on the south and west the maximum extent of Jumano territory (Fig. 11). Furthermore, the time period represented (ca. A.D. 1450–1600) terminates too early to allow any thought of identifying it with the Jumanos. Occasional Perdiz Pointed Stem points appear in peripheral components of the focus, apparently late, but these obviously represent intrusives from the Toyah Focus to the south and west.

The Nueces Focus

Along the Nueces canyon in Edwards, Real, and Uvalde counties occur late archaeological sites designated "Mound B" and "Kitchen Midden" cultures by Huskey (1935:105–14). "Mound B" culture is characterized by rare conical, burned-rock mounds containing large numbers of small arrowpoints, principally of the type here called Eddy Expanding Stem (Plate 9; see Huskey 1935: Plate 15, No. 164, second and third from left), together with "a few scrapers," "rough bone crushers," "a combination knife and punch," and on the surface "a few potsherds, tempered with bone." Rare animal bones, principally those of deer, turkey, and small animals were found, but bison bones, artifacts of shell, large projectile points, and large knives were lacking. Two burials were found in "Mound B" sites; both were extended inhumations with associated artifacts. Artifacts found with the burials included numbers of small arrowpoints of types occurring in the mounds, carved shell pendants, carved stone plaques, and one thin finely chipped knife. The burials were covered with stone slabs, among which were found manos and metates, rubbing stones, and hammerstones.

"Kitchen Midden" sites were characterized by thin campsite debris in which occurred many bones of bison and deer, a rough black sand-tempered pottery, a reddish-gray bone-tempered pottery, sidescrapers and snub-nosed scrapers, double-pointed beveled flint knives ("of the common type"), and small arrowpoints. Among the arrowpoints illustrated are the type here called Perdiz Pointed Stem (Huskey 1935: Plate 15, No. 165, second from right), a side-and-base-notched point (Huskey 1935: Plate 15,

No. 165, right), and an unnamed side-notched point type (Huskey 1935: Plate 15, No. 165, central two points). The latter type is often basally notched and serrated. It resembles in outline the larger Frio Flared Stem points (Huskey 1935: Plate 14, No. 161, central two specimens) of the Uvalde Focus of the Nueces River region, and ranges in size from that of small arrowpoints to that of the smaller Frio Flared points. It is also quite similar to Scallorn Stemmed of this report (Plate IX*f*), and is probably the typological prototype of the latter.

Excavations and survey work of the University of Texas have not demonstrated the validity of these complexes as separate cultures, but future work may yet do so. At the present time all of the late pottery and small arrowpoint sites of the Nueces canyon are grouped together to form the Nueces Focus. Diagnostics are Eddy Stemmed points together with the diminutive Frio Stemmed, or proto-Scallorn Stemmed points, bone- and sand-tempered pottery (possibly Doss Redware; see note 5, this chapter), snub-nosed scrapers, double-pointed knives, finely chipped blades, flake drills with flake or discoidal bases, and probably flake knives.[2] The Perdiz Pointed Stem points, which occur rarely in components of this focus, are probably intrusives from the Toyah Focus to the north and east.

The Nueces Focus is found not only in the Nueces canyon and immediately adjacent areas, but likewise over an undefined area of the Coastal Plain to the south and west, including the Anacacho Mountain region and perhaps extending to the vicinity of Eagle Pass on the southwest. In excavated sites it appears to be the most recent of three prehistoric foci (the oldest is unidentified; the middle is Uvalde; Huskey 1935:108–9). If Huskey's classification is correct, and if the diminutive Frio-like points actually developed out of the earlier Frio Flared Stem points, the Nueces Focus may be regarded as a development out of the Uvalde Focus[3] under the influence of the Toyah Focus (represented by the intrusive Perdiz Pointed Stem points, and perhaps by the thin, red, bone-tempered pottery [Doss Redware?]).

In view of the known chronological position and distribution of the Nueces Focus, it could very well represent the archaeological culture of the Eagle Pass division of the Jumanos. However, it has not been found at all to the north and west, and hence falls far short of approximating the full Jumano range. If the Nueces Focus proves to be the archaeological culture of the Eagle Pass Jumanos, the distinction between this group and the Jumanos of Juan Sabeata would seem to be demonstrated.

The Austin Focus

Along the Colorado River above and below Austin, Texas, and in adjacent tributary areas, occur many late sites containing pottery and small arrowpoints in quantity. Analysis of collections from these sites reveals that they represent varying admixtures of two complexes. One of these is the Toyah Focus, and the other, the Austin Focus. The Austin Focus is very closely related to the Nueces Focus, and the two may well be merged when a more detailed knowledge of their respective complexes is obtained. There is some reason for believing that the Nueces Focus represents a developmental form of the Austin Focus.

Krieger and I identified the Austin Focus independently. While it has been described by Krieger (1946:165–68), his description is based on mixed Austin-Toyah foci sites, as well as pure Austin Focus components, and his western boundary of the focus is thereby over-extended. Both Krieger and I agree that the late dating of the focus, together with its range, suggest that it is the archaeological culture of the Tonkawa Indians of the late seventeenth and eighteenth centuries, whose distribution it parallels in detail.

The Austin Focus occurs primarily in the area extending from Abilene on the north to the Austin region on the south, including the valley of the Colorado River and immediately adjacent tributary drainages, the country lying between the Colorado and Brazos rivers, and part of the Brazos River Valley itself.[4] It is characterized by Eddy Stemmed Points, Scallorn Stemmed points, double-pointed beveled knives, large snub-nosed scrapers, finely chipped blades, flake knives, drills with flake bases, flint handaxes, Leon Plain pottery,[5] plain or engraved beads of bird leg bone, and burial in flexed position under cairns of stone slabs. Manos and some bone tools may be included in this complex, and intrusive pottery from the Frankston and Allen foci occurs in some quantity in the mixed Toyah-Austin foci sites of the Colorado River drainage, indicating both contemporaneity and trade relations with these foci.

If the Austin Focus is identified with the historic and protohistoric Tonkawa Indians, as seems indicated, then it is in all probability not the culture of the Jumanos. Certainly a Jumano identification for the focus is barred by its complete absence from most of the historic Jumano territory. However, another and supplementary identification may be suggested. The Tonkawa do not appear, by that name, in the historic records prior to the closing decade of the seventeenth century. Correlation of mixed Austin-Toyah foci with both the Allen Focus and the earlier Frankston Focus, on the other hand, suggests a much earlier appearance of the Austin Focus. In this connection it will be recalled that during the latter half of the seventeenth century, the Jumanos were consistently reported in association with the Cibola Indians, whose rancherias were located along the Colorado River. The Cibolas, therefore, may be tentatively identified with the Austin Focus and with the later Tonkawa Indians.

12
The Toyah and Livermore Foci

Components of the Toyah Focus are known from the Trans-Pecos area, the Pecos River, the Llano River drainage, the middle Colorado River, and the Brazos River in Hill County, Texas. In addition, the diagnostic point type, Perdiz Pointed Stem, occurs widely in surface collections. In this regard, however, it should be noted that other foci in Texas utilized Perdiz Pointed Stem points (Fig. 10), hence the distribution of the point type does not delineate the territory of the Toyah Focus alone. The nature of the focus and its original position can best be established by considering some of the known components.

The Lehmann Rockshelter

This shelter is located on the Charlie Lehmann ranch about three miles northeast of Doss, Gillespie County, Texas. It lies in the bluffs along the north side of Onion Creek, just above its junction with Threadgill Creek. The shelter is open to the southwest but is well protected by nearby hillsides (Plate V*A*). The surrounding region is rough, hilly terrain, covered with a thick growth of juniper, post-oak, live-oak, mesquite, and other vegetation, including lush stands of grasses in the clearings. Many pools of water stand against the tilted strata that form the floor of Onion and Threadgill creeks, and the flow of these small streams is seldom interrupted. Deer and turkey are still abundant in the region. Many burned-rock middens and campsites, largely attributable to the Round Rock and Uvalde foci, occur in the vicinity.[1]

The rockshelter itself is roughly crescentic in form (Plate VI*A*), measuring approximately 240 feet in length and ranging in depth from 4 to

60 feet. Most of the area beneath the overhang, however, is covered by heavy rock fall, leaving an area about 145 feet long and 9 to 20 feet wide along the back wall which contained alluvial and cultural deposits. The overhanging roof averages about 8 to 12 feet in height (Plate V*B*), and the surface of the deposits lies about ten feet above normal stream level, sloping some 7 feet from western to eastern end (Plate VI*b*). The maximum depth of deposits in the excavated area was 85 inches.

Along 138 feet of the rear wall and ceiling (Plate V*B*), pictographs are visible. These include conventionalized human figures, deer, birds, circles, circles with dots, parallel lines, long wavy or zigzag lines, dot designs (Plate V*C*), and design elements resembling the stacked rain cloud designs of the Southwest. Most of the pictographs are in red, although black and white pigments are represented.[2] It proved impossible to assign the authorship of the pictographs to any one complex.

Shallow circular mortar holes are present in the fallen "table rocks" at the front of the occupied area (Plate VI*A*). At the southeastern end of the shelter, Onion Creek runs beneath the overhang, thus providing a readily available and protected source of water.

Excavations

Excavations were made between December 31, 1935, and January 15, 1936, under the direction of A. M. Woolsey, field archaeologist for the Department of Anthropology, University of Texas. Work was begun at the southeastern edge of the area (Plate VI*A*) and progressed toward the northwest. Where possible, a vertical exposure of the deposits was maintained across the entire width of the excavated area. Toward the close of the investigations work shifted to the northwestern edge of the shelter. All alluvium of promise was excavated.

A contour map of the site was made prior to excavation. The provenience of all artifacts was recorded by (1) depth from the surface, (2) the day of work on which the specimen was discovered, and hence the approximate horizontal location (Fig. 13), and (3), very rarely, by the strata in which they were found. Single-point cross-sections of the stratigraphy were made at irregular intervals, but no effort was made to relate these isolated cross-sections to each other or to the general stratigraphy of the site. Nevertheless, a fairly clear picture of the stratigraphy emerges from a close inspection of the isolated cross-sections, the general field notes, and the numerous photographs. A reconstruction of this stratigraphy is presented in Figures 12 and 13, and Plate VI*B*.

In all, 395 specimens were brought in from the field, but stratigraphic data of any sort were available on only 261 artifacts, full data on even fewer. Many flint chips, and numerous fragments of animal bone,

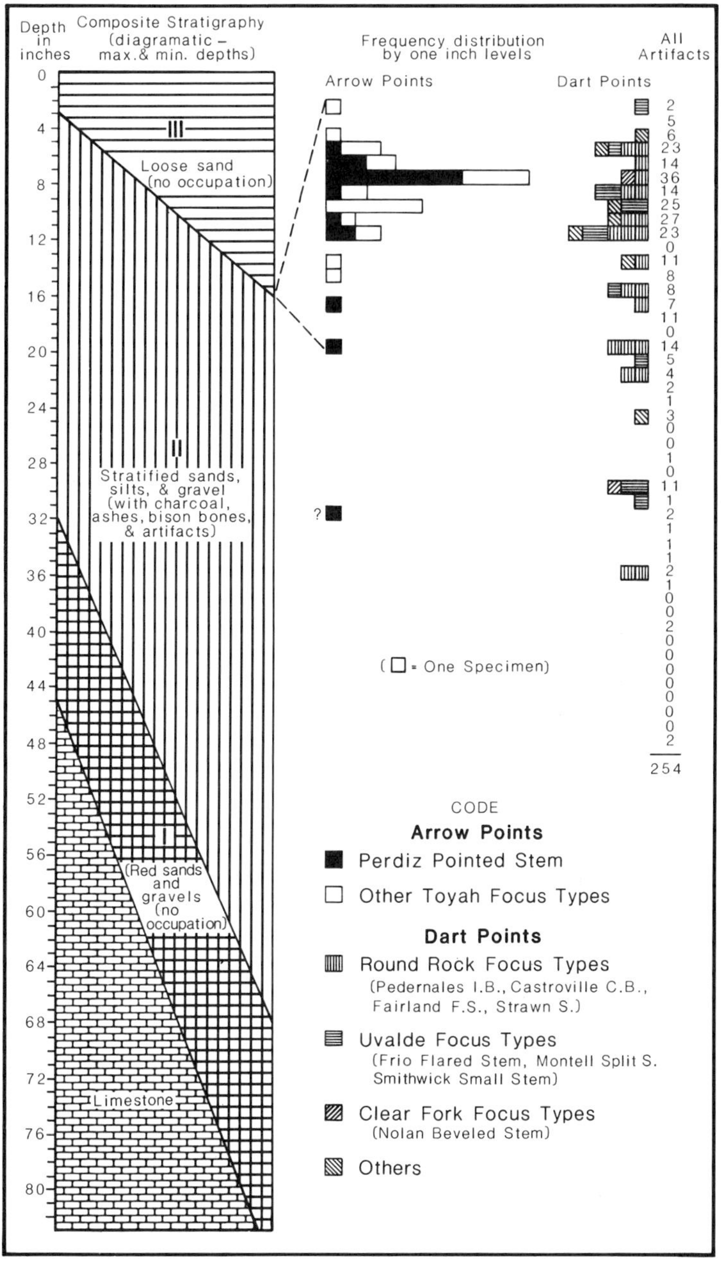

Figure 12. Stratigraphic distribution of projectile points in the Lehmann rockshelter.

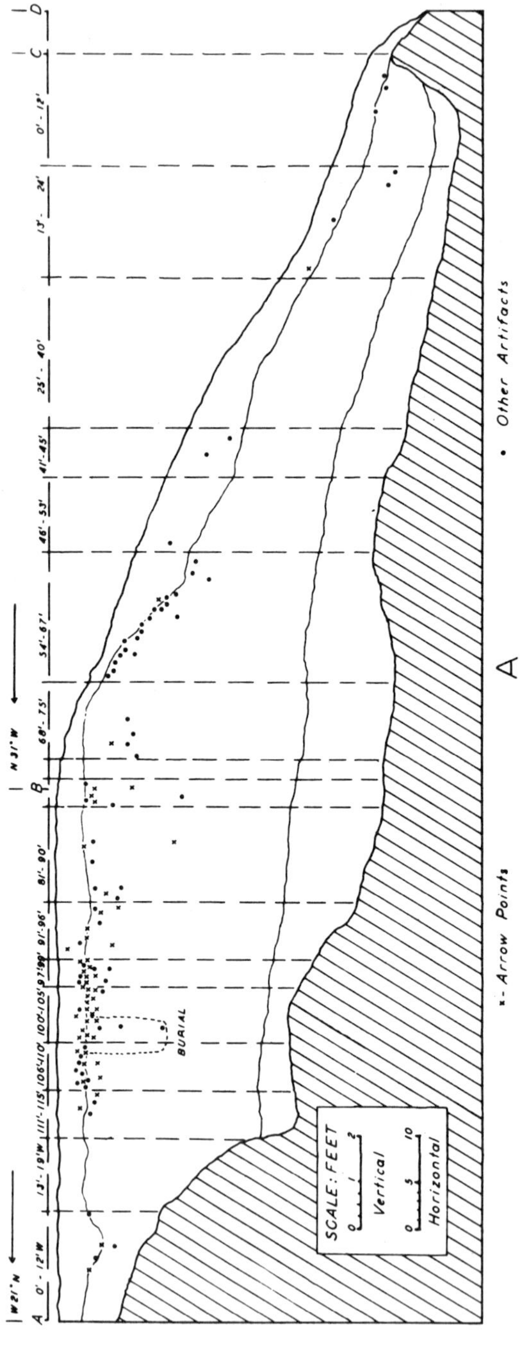
SCALE: FEET
Vertical
Horizontal
BURIAL
x - Arrow Points
• Other Artifacts
A
N 31' W
W 21' N

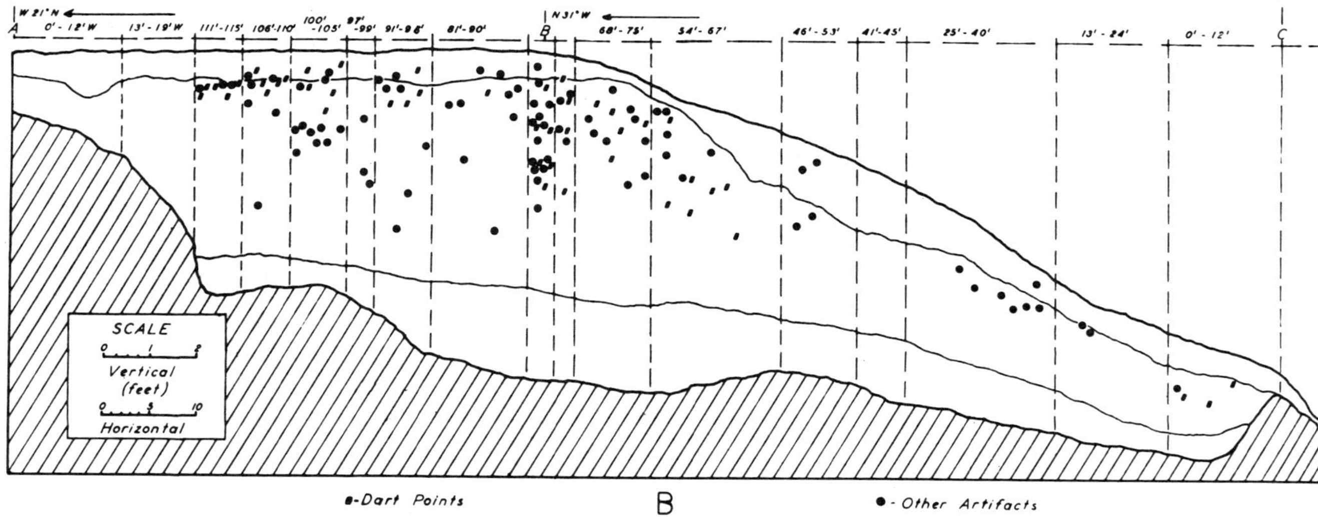

Figure 13. Stratigraphic distribution of all artifacts in the Lehmann rockshelter.

"apparently those of the buffalo," were recovered, and one human burial was excavated (Plate V*D*).

Stratigraphy

Three major stratigraphic units and many minor strata were apparent in the alluvial deposits of the shelter (Plate VI*B*). The uppermost of these units (III) consisted of loose sand containing much dung of domesticated animals. No artifacts were found in this stratum. The second and underlying unit (II) was a composite stratum of stratified sands, silts, and gravels containing much sand and charcoal, flint chips, artifacts, and broken animal bones. A human burial was found in the upper part of this stratum toward the northwestern edge of the deposits (Plate VI*A* and Fig. 13). A concentration of cultural debris, apparently representing the last aboriginal occupation of the site, here attributed primarily to the Toyah Focus, was noted at the very surface of this stratum. Lying directly on the bedrock floor of the shelter was the oldest stratigraphic unit (I), comprising strata of red sand and gravel with beds of silt represented locally. No artifacts or other indications of human occupation, except for a few fragments of charcoal, were found in this stratum. Maximum and minimum depths of strata are indicated diagramatically in Figure 12, and a reconstruction of the stratigraphic profile along section A-B-C-D (Plate VI*A*) is presented in Plate II.

Cultural Composition

Two of the artifacts recovered were potsherds, five were bone, and all other artifacts were made of stone, principally flint or chert. Out of the total of 261 artifacts, 93 were classed as projectile points. Large, rather roughly chipped points, called "dart points" here, made up 46 of the total, while the remaining 47 specimens were small thin points, often delicately chipped, made from thin flint flakes. These specimens are termed "arrowpoints." Because of their numbers and variability, and with due regard to the fact that most of the specimens in question belonged to types identified in previous work, projectile points were used as index fossils in analyzing the cultural composition and stratigraphy of the site.

The methodological procedure was as follows. All artifacts were divided into broad classes or categories, based on materials, and on general form and assumed function (i.e., projectile points, scrapers, metates, pottery). In each class of specimens, where sufficient numbers were available, a further subdivision into types, or stylistic groups, was made.[3] A composite profile of the shelter deposits was constructed, and on it the location of all specimens in each type was plotted. Depth and approximate horizontal position together with available stratigraphic data, were used in plotting specimen location. Certain conclusions were at once evident:

1) All arrowpoints, with one exception, occurred in the upper part of Stratum II at depths of less than 20 inches, and only five of the 47 specimens were found below 12 inches in depth (Fig. 12). Most of them appeared to cluster about the surface of Stratum II, primarily in the northwestern portion of the excavated area (Fig. 13), a conclusion borne out by such stratigraphic notes as are available.
2) Conversely, dart points were more evenly distributed throughout the upper two thirds of Stratum II (Figs. 12 and 13), and occurred at absolutely greater depths than the arrowpoints.
3) The stratigraphic position of the human burial indicated that it probably belonged with the late camp marked by the concentration of arrowpoints (Fig. 13).
4) Apparently, at least two cultural complexes were represented: a dart point complex present throughout the occupation of the site, and an arrowpoint complex present only during the more recent period of occupation. There was apparently, but not indisputably, an overlap in the occupation of the cave by peoples possessing the two complexes. That is, people using arrowpoints first appeared in the shelter while others using dart points still inhabited the site or the region, or at best very little time separated the two occupations. It is of course possible that the occupants of the shelter simply took over or invented the use of arrowpoints without the intervention of new occupants at all.

These tentative conclusions indicated that further methodological procedure was necessary.

Inasmuch as arrowpoints were found almost entirely in the upper 12 to 18 inches of the deposits, other artifacts restricted to this same stratigraphic position probably would represent additional elements of the arrowpoint complex. The combination of types found exclusively, or almost exclusively, in the upper 12 to 18 inches was immediately recognizable as characteristic of the Toyah Focus (Plate VII). In those instances where the stratigraphic position of artifacts of this complex was given in the notes in addition to recording by depth and horizontal position, the specimens were found to occur in the upper few inches of Stratum II, or at its surface, confirming the position of the Toyah Focus in the deposits.

Conversely, artifact types found throughout the occupational strata would probably represent other elements of the dart point complex. Artifacts of these types, therefore, were grouped into a second complex, one recognizable as the Edwards Plateau Aspect of the Balcones Phase, an archaic food-gathering culture widely distributed in Texas (Kelley 1940; Kelley et al. 1940:30–31). Diagnostic artifacts, principally dart point types of two complexes of this culture already discussed, the Round Rock and

Uvalde foci, were present in some numbers, and three artifacts of types attributed to the Clear Fork Focus of the aspect were found. Still other types present cannot as yet be referred with assurance to any focus.

The Toyah Focus Component

Artifacts attributable to the Toyah Focus in the Lehmann rockshelter include arrowpoints of the types Perdiz Pointed Stem, Clinton Contracting Stem, "Form 63," and Fresno Triangular Blade. Other arrowpoint types represented are Scallorn Stemmed of the Austin Focus, Piedras Triple Notched, and Saucita Split Base of the Bravo Valley Aspect, and others of types whose cultural provenance is as yet uncertain (Plate VII*a-i*).

Additional artifacts of the Toyah Focus from Lehmann shelter are snub-nosed scrapers, small awls or drills with discoidal flake bases, double-pointed blades or knives with slightly beveled alternate edges, many lanceolate, squat triangular, elongated triangular, and small triangular blades, usually well chipped, and tubular bone beads (Plate VII*j-u*). Other elements of the culture (not illustrated) are thin potsherds with sand and bone temper and a red-washed polished surface (Doss Redware), large crudely chipped choppers, hammerstones, "spokeshaves" (large flakes with small crescentic concave scraping areas on one edge), bone awls, and one eyeless fish-bone needle. In Plate VI*C* the relative frequency of these artifacts is plotted diagramatically by type or class, and the actual frequency of each type is shown, while their approximate horizontal and vertical distribution is plotted in Fig. 13.

As previously indicated, the human burial probably belongs with the Toyah Focus component. The skeleton itself did not survive disinterment; the physical type is therefore unknown. This is extremely unfortunate, as this is the only burial discovered which can be referred to the Toyah Focus, and probably to the Jumano Indians, with any assurance at all. According to the field notes, the skeleton was that of a young adult female. The body had been placed in the grave in a loosely flexed position, lying on its right side with knees drawn up and legs flexed, arms folded loosely on the chest, face turned to the north, and the head resting on and supported by a small boulder (Plate V*D*). The axis of the body was oriented roughly east-west with the head at the east. The tubular bone bead shown in Plate VII*n* lay at the left ankle or on the left foot; no other artifacts were associated.

The floor of the grave in the upper part of Stratum II was 30 inches beneath the surface. Large stones had been placed on edge around the head and at the foot of the burial within the grave. A large stone slab lay over the body, and over this were tilted two other large slabs. The upper ends of these slabs must have protruded from the top of Stratum II, although there are no photographs or notes available to prove or disprove this statement.

This type of flexed burial in a stone-protected grave in or near the campsite with little or no mortuary furniture is also characteristic of the Edwards Plateau Aspect, the Austin Focus, other late complexes as well.

The Edwards Plateau Aspect Component

Dart points from Stratum II belong, as previously stated, to types thought to be diagnostic of the Round Rock, Uvalde, and Clear Fork foci of the Edwards Plateau Aspect. Other dart points, including specimens classed as Yarbrough Stemmed, Bluffton Barbed, Bulverde Barbed (Plate VIII*h-j*), and unidentified types (not shown), perhaps belong with one or more of these foci but cannot yet be referred to any of them. One fragmentary specimen, which is not shown, is representative of either Bracken Broad Base of the Morhiss Focus of the lower Guadalupe River, or else Juno Broad Base of the Pecos River Focus.

Dart points of types characteristic of the Round Rock Focus include specimens of Pedernales Indented Base, Strawn Stemmed, Fairland Flared Stem (Plate VIII*a, e, c* respectively), and Castroville Convex Base (not shown). Diagnostic types of the Uvalde Focus present in the site include specimens of Smithwick Small Stem, Frio Flared Stem, and Montell Split Stem (Plate VIII*b, d, f*). The Clear Fork Focus[4] was represented by two specimens of Nolan Beveled Stem (Plate VIII*g*), as well as by one specimen of a Clear Fork Gouge (Plate VIII*l, m,* reverse and obverse side).

Other artifacts of this complex were common items of the Edwards Plateau Aspect in general, rather than representing diagnostic traits of individual foci. These include large and irregularly shaped blades with crude chipping, crudely chipped spike-like blades, fairly well chipped triangular blades, large flake sidescrapers, small percussion-chipped choppers made from cores (ranging into rejects and modified nodules), and one-hand unshaped (one shaped specimen) manos, either single or double faced, all shown in Plate VIII. One specimen, best described as a "chipped celt," was found; and other specimens belonging to this complex, but not illustrated here, include fragments of oval-bowl metates (or seed slabs), large flakes with small drill points or "gravers," heavy pick-like blades crudely chipped from cores, and one large stemmed knife.

The relative frequency of artifacts assigned to this focus is illustrated graphically by type or class in Plate VI*C* and in Figure 13; the approximate vertical and horizontal distribution of the specimens of this complex in the shelter deposits is given.

Chronology

There can be no doubt of the relative chronological position of the Toyah Focus with regard to the Edwards Plateau Aspect in the Lehmann rockshelter. As previously pointed out, the Edwards Plateau Aspect was represented throughout the upper two-thirds of Stratum II, while the

Toyah Focus appeared in the shelter only at the very close of the same depositional period. If the one Perdiz point recorded at a depth of 32 inches actually came from that depth, there may have been contact between the Toyah Focus and the Edwards Plateau Aspect at an early period in the shelter's occupation, and a correspondingly greater overlap between the two cultures in time. In view of the inadequate stratigraphic data given for individual specimens, it does not seem wise to place too much emphasis on the evidence of one specimen.

Nevertheless, there was apparently an overlap between the late Edwards Plateau occupation and the Toyah Focus as shown by the distribution of arrowpoints and dart points in Figure 12. This is important, if true, and the bulk of the evidence here and in other sites indicates that such an overlap probably occurred. Nevertheless, in this site the evidence is insufficient to prove the point. Thus, much of the apparent overlap in distribution of dart points and arrowpoints probably results from lack of sufficient stratigraphic control. It is emphasized in the field notes that the surface of Stratum II varied greatly in depth from front to back of the shelter, yet with rare exceptions the stratigraphic sections were made in the center of the transverse exposure only. This accounts for the apparent occurrence of specimens in Stratum II (Fig. 13), when as a matter of fact none were found there. This probably accounts for much, if not all, of the apparent overlap in occupation, but there is no way of checking the point.

Dart points of the various foci of the Edwards Plateau Aspect are represented in such small numbers that it is impossible to speak with assurance of their relative position in the strata (Fig. 12). Such evidence as is available would indicate that the Clear Fork, Uvalde, and Round Rock foci are of approximately the same age in this site. It is known from previous work that the Round Rock and Clear Fork foci existed side by side in the Colorado River drainage over a very long span of time. It is also known that in the Edwards Plateau region to the west of the Colorado, and especially along the Nueces River, there was an early Round Rock Focus occupation followed by the Uvalde Focus. While the Round Rock Focus in the west gave way to the Uvalde Focus, it survived until late prehistoric times in the Colorado River valley, and was thus contemporary with the Uvalde Focus during the later days of its own existence. This chronological picture is apparently reflected in the Edwards Plateau Aspect levels in Lehmann rockshelter, which is located in a geographically intermediate position between east and west.

The presence of Uvalde Focus artifacts in the lower occupation levels at this site indicates that the older occupation here is relatively recent in terms of central Texas archaeology. The Toyah Focus in Lehmann rockshelter, therefore, represents a very late occupation indeed, but since there is no trace of historic contact in the site, the late prehistoric period is probably represented. There is no evidence in the shelter that allows the assignment of actual dates to any of the complexes represented. Again, it is worthy of note that the occupation of the shelter coincided with all but the earliest and most recent stages of alluvial deposition there and presumably elsewhere along the stream, though the latter point requires demonstration. This is in keeping with evidence from elsewhere in the state, as will soon become evident.

Buzzard Cave

Buzzard Cave is located on the Brazos River in Hill County, Texas. It was discovered and has been partially excavated by Robert L. Stephenson in connection with the river valley surveys administered by the Smithsonian Institution. Stephenson kindly allowed me to make reference to his unpublished discoveries at this site.

The cave, in my opinion, is almost a pure Toyah Focus component. A total of 54 arrowpoints were found, and of these 30 were representative of the type Perdiz Pointed Stem. Also found there were snub-nosed scrapers, for the most part smaller than the customary Toyah Focus specimens, double-pointed beveled knives, small drills or awls, flake knives or scrapers, and a few potsherds, principally plain red and brown ware (apparently Doss Redware and Leon Plain). Finely chipped blades were apparently rare at the site, and mussel shell was present in some quantity in place of the bison bone of the Lehmann rockshelter. Notably present was one obsidian arrow or dart point of unfamiliar type. Because obsidian is obtainable no closer than New Mexico or northern Mexico, this is indicative of widespread trade relations. The northern position of the site geographically, and the freedom from admixture with cultures such as the Austin Focus, suggest that a fairly early component of the Toyah Focus is represented, although no data as to the actual age of the site were obtained. It should be noted that the site is located along the shortest route from the Concho River (probably the "Rio Nueces" of the Spanish documents) to the Tejas towns of the east.

Middle Colorado River Components

Along the Colorado River from south of Austin northward to at least beyond the mouth of the Llano River, occur numerous late sites, usually superimposed on burned-rock middens of the Clear Fork and Round Rock foci or present in the upper levels of these. Most of these sites are mixed components of the Austin and Toyah foci, although some nearly pure Austin Focus sites have been noted. Furthermore, in these sites occur trade wares from east Texas cultures such as the late prehistoric Frankston Focus and the early historic Allen Focus, attributed to the Hasinai Indians.

One of these sites, Fall Creek Site No. 3 has been discussed in print (Jackson 1938b).

Fall Creek Site No. 3

Judging by the artifacts described, this site is basically a component of the Round Rock and Clear Fork foci with admixtures of other related cultures. However, there is also a late occupation principally attributable to the Toyah and Austin foci. A total of 111 arrowpoints were found and 80 of these came from Midden No. 2. Seventy-one of the 80 points came from the upper 12 inches of the deposits, although dart points occurred to depths of 39 inches, and no arrowpoints were found deeper than 23 inches (Jackson 1938b:84–88).

Pottery also was found in unusually large quantities in these middens, principally in the levels producing arrowpoints. The ware which Jackson calls Coahuiltecan is that here called Doss Redware. Snub-nosed scrapers, fine drills, well-chipped blades, and double-pointed beveled knives were found in the site, but from Jackson's description it is impossible to say definitely that they were associated with the pottery and arrowpoints. It is important to note that four artifacts of European origin came from the upper levels of Midden No. 2, a piece of lead at a depth of 1 inch, a section of brass (bearing the inscription "Anheuser Busch, St. Louis") at 18 inches, a silver U.S. quarter dollar (dated 1876) at 9 inches, and a blue trade bead at 14 inches. Jackson notes the possibility of recent intrusion of some of these specimens but notes that the trade bead is similar to those found in historic sites (Allen Focus) in east Texas, from which trade sherds are likewise present (Jackson 1938b:115–16).

Other Components

It is unnecessary to discuss in detail other Toyah Focus components along the Colorado River. They invariably show some admixture with the Austin Focus, and they are invariably late, although evidence of actual historic contact is usually scanty and indirect, or actually lacking. All of them occur in the upper part of the so-called "twenty-foot terrace" of the Colorado River, the more recent of two alluvial terraces assigned to the Recent epoch (Kelley 1947). All of them represent an occupation which either immediately followed that of the Round Rock and Clear Fork foci, or, more often, mingled with the later phases of these complexes. The association with Allen and Frankston foci trade wares occurs in several instances.

Pecos River Components of the Toyah Focus

I have made collections from eroding sites along the Pecos River between Girvin and Iraan, and much farther to the south just above the Pecos canyon, and have described some of these sites in Kelley et al. (1940:90–91). The complexes represented are typically of Toyah Focus affiliation, although referred to as the Wichita Phase at the time the collections were made. Again, the age of the sites is very late, since they are included in the upper part of the most recent alluvial formation, and in this instance almost pure Toyah Focus components are represented.

Trans-Pecos Components

Many of the sites found by the Peabody Museum-Sul Ross College Big Bend expedition and referred to as the Bravo Valley Aspect at this date prove to belong to the Toyah Focus. Alpine 9:12 and Alpine 9:13 are located in the Elephant Mountain region south of Alpine, Texas. The artifact inventory from these sites shows a predominantly Toyah Focus affiliation, with the addition of manos and metates to the complex (Kelley et al. 1940:119–20). Other such sites are found throughout the Trans-Pecos region, although none have been excavated. Again, the Toyah Focus components in this region occur in the most recent strata of the valley alluvium, although no historical associations have been noted.

The Toyah Focus Summary and Discussion

The Toyah Focus is almost exactly the complex required to satisfy the criteria of Jumano archaeological culture. It has a general artifact complex sufficiently similar to that of the Bravo Valley Aspect to indicate close relationship. The diagnostic point type, Perdiz Pointed Stem, is likewise one of the dominant types of the Bravo Valley Aspect. Interestingly enough, this is also the dominant point type of the Frankston Focus, the prehistoric culture of the Hasinai Indians with whom the Jumanos maintained trade relations, and of the Rockport Focus of the Gulf Coast in the vicinity of Corpus Christi.[5] Furthermore, actual examples of Bravo Valley Aspect artifacts have been found in Toyah Focus components in central Texas (Piedras Triple Notched and Saucita Split Base arrowpoints in Lehmann rockshelter; also one example of a Bravo Valley type arrowshaft straightener from Mason County; and Frankston-Allen foci artifacts—Patton Engraved and related pottery types—in Colorado River components). The complex belongs chronologically to the late prehistoric and early historic periods, although actual instances of the occurrence of historic artifacts in Toyah Focus components are rare and not too well documented. The requisite type of culture is present, and the geographical range of the Toyah Focus is very nearly identical with that of the Jumanos.

However, the identification of the Toyah Focus with the Jumano Indians is not completely in accord with all of the distributional evidence. No Toyah Focus sites have been located in the critical Concho River drainage, supposedly the center of Jumano activities. This is not necessarily evidence to the contrary, but seems to be rather of the nature of negative evidence. Several weekend field trips to the vicinity of San Angelo resulted in the discovery of very few sites of any kind. No arrowpoint-bearing sites were located, although snub-nosed scrapers and flake knives were found in several sites eroding from the surface of plowed fields. No collections of arrowpoints, or even of dart points, in quantity were located in this area. Consequently, there is no evidence as to the nature of the late cultures of the Concho River. This lack of late sites is disturbing and suggests that the archaeologist would do well not to accept the identification of the "Rio Nueces" with the modern-day Concho River as completely settled and assured, in view of the fact that more southerly streams, such as the Llano River, do have Toyah Focus components in some numbers.*

Furthermore, the Toyah Focus is notably lacking in the sand dune region running southeastward from the corner of New Mexico, an area in which Jumano occupation might have been anticipated. However, the sand dune country may have been Apache territory in the early historic period, and the Jumano territory may have been farther to the east or more likely to the west along the Pecos River. Unfortunately, the Toyah Focus has not been reported from the campsites along Toyah Creek itself, and Toyah Creek is another of the areas in which the Jumanos were centered during the early historic period.

Whatever the facts regarding the early historic period, however, the Toyah Focus is the only known culture which in any way meets the criteria of a Jumano archaeological culture. If we confine the comparison to that of Jumano distribution in the seventeenth century most of the difficulties disappear. This suggests that the Toyah Focus is indeed the archaeological culture of the seventeenth and early eighteenth century Jumanos, but that the archaeological culture of the earlier Jumanos was something else again. It has already been suggested that the early historic Jumanos of the Pecos River and southeastern New Mexico possessed a Bravo Valley Aspect culture. There is, however, another possibility. Sites of the sand dune region of southeastern New Mexico and adjacent sections of Texas are rich in artifacts of the Livermore Focus, and, interestingly enough, typical arrowpoints of Livermore Focus types have been reported from the

---

*Recent field work in the Concho River area has produced Perdiz Pointed Stem points in quantity. (J.C.K.)

campsites along Toyah Creek. A discussion of the Livermore Focus, as the possible archaeological culture of the early historic Jumanos is therefore in order.

The Livermore Focus

This complex has been described in Kelley et al. (1940) but has not yet received thorough investigation of any sort. Open campsites and rock-shelters are the typical sites. Artifacts include easily recognizable small arrowpoints such as Livermore Barbed, Livermore Serrate, and Toyah Triple Notched (Plate IX*g*); snub-nosed scrapers, double-pointed knives, small graver points, flake knives, finely chipped blades, small shaft straighteners of *malpais* stone, slab metates, and one-hand manos. Pottery and permanent houses are lacking and there is no indication of the practice of agriculture. This is the oldest known Big Bend culture possessing the bow and arrow and associated items. In the Trans-Pecos, Livermore Focus components are often mixed with early Chisos Focus and late Pecos River Focus components. The stratigraphic position of sites noted *in situ* in valley alluvium places the culture in the period of erosion immediately preceding the deposition of the Kokernot Formation of the Big Bend. Known sites of the Bravo Valley Aspect and the Toyah Focus occur in the overlying Kokernot Formation itself (Kelley et al. 1940; Albritton and Bryan 1939).[6]

Characteristic Livermore Focus points have been found in New Mexico under circumstances suggesting a date of around A.D. 900 (Haury 1936a: Plate 18*e*),[7] a date in keeping with the stratigraphic position of the complex in the Big Bend. In southeastern New Mexico, Mera found typical Livermore points in both "Midden Circles" and "Camp Sites," in association with local sand-tempered brown wares and intrusive Southwestern wares such as El Paso Polychrome and Chupadero Black-on-White (Mera 1938:13–23, and Plate 3*A*, fourth from left, upper row, and *B*, third from left, upper row). In the adjoining sand dune belt of Texas, artifacts of the Livermore Focus occur in large numbers, and there is again an apparent association with Southwestern pottery of the types noted above. This suggests that in this general region the Livermore Focus survived into, and perhaps through, the A.D. 1200–1600 period. The approximate distribution of the Livermore Focus is given in Figure 10.

The principal difference between the Toyah and Livermore foci lies in point type and pottery type. The general stone complex is very similar. The distribution of the focus is suggestive of the distribution of the Jumanos in the late sixteenth and early seventeenth centuries. Furthermore, typical Livermore points are reported from the campsites along Toyah Creek which probably are to be attributed to the Jumanos of 1583 (Kelley 1933;

see also Kelley 1937). This suggests that the Livermore Focus may well have been the archaeological culture of the early historic Jumanos. However, if this is true, the early Jumanos cannot have had a Bravo Valley Aspect type of culture, and there are likewise objections to such an identification in terms of the general Texas archaeological picture. Further work will be needed to resolve the question.

Jumano and Patarabueye Archaeology: Summary and Conclusions

The archaeological culture of the Patarabueye Indians can be identified with assurance as the Bravo Valley Aspect, in particular the Concepción and Conchos foci of that aspect. This culture appeared at around A.D. 1200 and evolved *in situ* along the Rio Grande and Rio Conchos near La Junta, finally merging into the historic Spanish-American occupation in the nineteenth century.

The archaeological culture of the Jumano Indians is less certainly but quite probably identifiable with the Toyah Focus of central and Trans-Pecos Texas. The culture is that of a hunting group related to the Bravo Valley Aspect but distinct in detail. The distribution of this culture and the other pertinent factors identify it with fair assurance as the archaeological culture of the Jumanos of the late seventeenth and early eighteenth centuries. The Toyah Focus, on the other hand, may prove to be absent in those areas occupied by the Jumanos of the fifteenth and sixteenth centuries, and the archaeological culture of the Jumanos of that period may alternatively be identifiable with either the Bravo Valley Aspect itself, or with the Livermore Focus.

In the following section an attempt will be made to relate the data derived from historical sources to those based on archaeological studies, and from this composite approach to clarify the general picture of Jumano and Patarabueye identity and relationship.

13
Ethnic and Cultural Differentiation of the Jumanos and Patarabueyes

Distinctive Histories

Archaeological and documentary data provide us with a relatively clear picture of the development of Patarabueye culture from about A.D. 1200 to near the end of the eighteenth century. Throughout that span of time their culture develops *in situ* in the La Junta region. Changes in culture appear from time to time and the influence of other cultures is clearly visible, especially Spanish influence after the end of the seventeenth century. Furthermore, from time to time, other groups may have been added to the Patarabueye nucleus. Nevertheless, there is definite continuity of culture throughout; individual village sites continued to be occupied from around A.D. 1200 until the present. It is a fair assumption that the original Patarabueye physical stock is still represented in dilute form in the modern villages of the region.

The appearance of the Patarabueyes in the historical records, either by that name or by the names of the constituent groups, is almost invariably in connection with the political and religious affairs of the Rio Grande and northern Mexico, and the tribes of that region. Almost never do any of the Patarabueye groups appear in connection with the affairs of the central Texas tribes and missions.

Jumano history is likewise fairly clear from 1583 to the first quarter of the eighteenth century. Uncertainty as to the archaeological culture of the early Jumanos makes it impossible to discuss their culture prior to that date. Throughout the span of Jumano history the name of the group appears repeatedly, not only in the political and religious affairs of the Rio Grande from La Junta to Isleta, New Mexico, but in those of central, southern, and eastern Texas as well. They appear in association with groups scattered over half of the area of Texas. In the early historic period they are often involved in the intrigues of the La Junta towns, but after 1690, as the Patarabueyes are slowly acculturated under Spanish influence, the Jumanos are rarely mentioned in the La Junta documents. Instead, they are noted in the records of the San Antonio missions and elsewhere in central Texas up until the time of their final absorption by the Apaches. Although they overlap, the respective histories of Jumanos and Patarabueyes are convincingly distinct.

Distinctive Territories

The distribution of the Jumanos (Fig. 1) and their archaeological culture (Fig. 10) is clearly distinct from that of the Patarabueyes (see Map). In the records I can find no reference to Patarabueye groups away from the Rio Grande-Rio Conchos drainage, with one exception. When the Teran-Massanet expedition encountered the Jumanos on the Guadalupe River in 1691, they listed among the tribes associated with the Jumanos the name "Chalome." This is probably a reference to the group known variously as Cholomes, Cholombos, and Chocolomes, and presumably should be included in the Patarabueye group (see Chapter 9, note 8). It should likewise be noted that the French spoke of "Palaquesson" or "Palaquechaune" Indians in southern Texas in contact with the Jumanos. "Palaquesson" conceivably could refer to the Polaques or Pulicos, one of the Patarabueye groups, but this is a rather imaginative connection. On the contrary, there are Patarabueye disclaimers of knowledge of the territory to the east of the Rio Grande.

The Jumanos, on the other hand, spoke freely of their travels in central, southern, and eastern Texas, and Sabeata declared in 1683 that the land occupied by the Jumanos lay six days' journey east of La Junta and three days' journey east of the buffalo plains (see Chapter 4). In this statement and others, La Junta is included in the Jumano range, but is specifically described as the winter residence only. The range of the Jumanos, therefore, overlaps that of the Patarabueyes in the west, but the two groups unquestionably claimed and occupied distinct territories.

Distinctive Cultures

In the concluding section of this study, detailed summaries of the respective Jumano and Patarabueye cultures are presented. It may be pointed out here, however, that there are certain clear and basic distinctions between the cultures. The Jumanos were wandering bison hunters and traders; the Patarabueyes were settled village-dwelling farmers. The Jumanos occupied temporary or movable "tents," obviously skin tipis of Plains type; the Patarabueyes lived in permanent earth lodges and in organized villages, complete with plazas and "streets." Detailed differences are apparent in the archaeological cultures. Pottery is of rare occurrence in the Toyah Focus, thought to be of Jumano origin, and the types represented are Doss Redware and Leon Plain. In the Concepción Focus (representing a comparable time period), pottery is of frequent occurrence and the common types are Chinati Plain, Neck-Banded, Striated, and Paloma Red-on-Gray, Capote Red-on-Brown, Capote Plain, and an unnamed polished red ware. In stone, the most notable difference is in arrowpoint type. The Patarabueyes of the Bravo Valley Aspect used arrowpoints of the types Perdiz Pointed Stem, Piedras Triple Notched, Frisco Base Notched, Saucita Split Base, Clinton Contracting Stem, Fresno Triangular, and minor types represented by only a few specimens in the collections. These types occur together constantly in Bravo Valley sites and in fairly consistent proportions. The Jumanos of the Toyah Focus used only Perdiz Pointed Stem, Clinton Contracting Stem, and Fresno Triangular. The side-notched and split base types of the Bravo Valley Aspect appear only sporadically, and then usually singly, in Toyah Focus sites. Many of the characteristic Bravo Valley Aspect artifacts—notched sinker stones, shaped manos and oval-bowl metates, carved stone bowls, "cloud blowers," specialized shaft straighteners, sandstone shaft abraders, certain types of specialized mortars and pestles—are completely lacking in known Toyah Focus components.

From the standpoint of the archaeologist, the Toyah Focus and the Bravo Valley Aspect, in particular the Concepción Focus of that aspect, are clearly distinct cultures. But can the archaeological concept of cultures be employed in the interpretation of the actual patterns of behavior concerned in this instance? We know that many, if not all, of the Jumanos spent their winters at La Junta. Why should bison hunters and traders take with them on a hunting trip of months' duration and many hundreds of miles distance such domestic items as net-sinkers, cloud blowers, and household ceramics? Obviously, on the buffalo hunt tipis would be of greater utility than earth lodges. Is it not possible to explain the difference between Jumano and Patarabueye culture entirely in terms of such factors? And if so, does not the entire distinction between Jumanos and Patarabueyes tend to disappear, leaving the alternate possibility that the Jumanos were specialized hunters, or members of a "hunt society" in the La Junta settlements?

This is at first glance a tempting hypothesis. But on closer inspection it is at once apparent that there are cultural distinctions between the two groups that cannot be disposed of in such an easy manner. Thus, it is difficult to explain why hunters departing on such a long journey would leave behind them the arrow-shaft straighteners and abraders needed in maintaining their weapons. Even harder to understand is the fact that arrowpoints representing only three of the six types used at La Junta, and found together repeatedly in house after house there, were carried by the hunters. And finally, pottery does occur in the Jumano archaeological sites, but the types represented differ from those of La Junta. Differences of this type appear to be explainable only in terms of historical factors affecting the relations existing between discrete cultures.

Thus, the Jumano and Patarabueye cultures were apparently autonomous patterns of living long established in their respective areas. The close relation that existed between them is probably to be explained in terms of a common origin, together with long continued contact. The distinctions that have been noted are best explained in terms of divergent developments resulting from their varied histories, contacts, and environments together with selective borrowing and perhaps some variations in the original parent cultures.

Jumanos and Patarabueyes in the Records

The use of the term Jumano, and its application to other groups in the historical records, requires further discussion. The simplest procedure would be to accept Scholes's interpretation of the term "Jumano" as signifying "tattooed" or "painted." Certainly the term seem to have been so used in New Mexico; the Havasupai, the eastern Pueblos and the Wichitas were called Jumanos in this sense. But if we apply the term in this restricted sense in western and central Texas the inadequacy of the usage is at once apparent. Practically all of the Indians of eastern, southern and central Texas, and probably those in the west as well, seem to have practiced tattooing or face painting to some degree. Among these certainly were the Tejas (Hasinai), the Tonkawas, and the Patarabueyes. Ironically, the followers of Sabeata were *not* definitely tattooed or painted; at least none of the references examined in this study mention painted or tattooed Jumanos. And yet when the followers of Sabeata were encountered in company with Tejas Indians, the term Jumano was applied to the former and not to the Tejas, who were definitely tattooed peoples. This discrepancy occurs repeatedly; Sabeata's followers are invariably called Jumanos, or some variation of this name, regardless of the company in which they are found, and the other tribes who accompany them are called by band or tribal names, rather than by the term Jumano, even when they are described as *rayados* Indians.

Whatever the circumstances in New Mexico, the term Jumano as used in Texas definitely referred to one group, the group whose history has been traced in detail in this study. It was used by both Spanish and French in referring to them, and by other Indians as well. Thus, La Salle was told by Indians of the lower Colorado River that their chief had been among the

"Chouman." The very fact that the French acquired the use of the name independently of the Spaniards and that they applied it in a varied phonetic form to one specific group and not to tattooed Indians in general is highly significant. But more than this, the Jumanos seem to have applied the term to themselves. At El Paso in 1680, Sabeata referred to his tribe as "the extended nation of the Humanas" if I have interpreted correctly his "Declaration." And again, it was not until he had talked at length with Sabeata, on the Guadalupe River in 1691, that Massanet commented that the "Chomas" under Sabeata were the Indians called "Jumanes" in New Mexico. Presumably, this information was derived from Sabeata himself.

Actually, the confusion of the Jumanos and the Patarabueyes in the historical sources is attributable almost entirely to Espejo, and to Obregón's paraphrase of the Espejo account. In view of the fact that Espejo's account was written from memory many months later, and that it is notably in error in other particulars, there seems no reason to allow this one statement to offset the weighty evidence to the contrary presented in previous pages. The distinction between Patarabueyes and Jumanos and the existence of a separate Jumano group seem amply demonstrated.

Linguistic Affiliation of the Jumanos and Patarabueyes

No new data regarding the linguistic affiliation of the Jumanos have been introduced. The Jumanos were closely related to the Patarabueyes, but did not necessarily speak the same language. The latter were probably of Uto-Aztecan affiliation, in view of their close relationship and proximity to the Conchos tribes. The Jumanos may likewise have belonged to this language group, but on the other hand, their language may have been the Caddoan of their close friends the Tejas, the Tonkawan of their central Texas friends and allies the Cibolas (if Cibola and Tonkawa are identical), the Coahuiltecan of their neighbors along the Guadalupe River, or the Athapascan of the Lipan Apaches with whom they finally merged. I can see no evidence pointing with any assurance to any one of these linguistic affiliations, and I judge that the entire question is likely to remain unsolved, unless new documentary material appears.

Part V
Summary and Conclusions

14
The Patarabueyes

Utilizing the materials presented in previous pages, with the addition of supplementary data of a comparative nature, trait lists have been compiled for the Jumano and Patarabueye cultures. Cultural elements and traits derived from documentary sources are indicated by the superscript "d" and those derived from archaeological sources by the superscript "a." In compiling the list, the Toyah Focus was accepted as the archaeological culture of the Jumanos, and the Bravo Valley Aspect as the archaeological culture of the Patarabueyes. The sources for this information can be found in other chapters, so I have not cited specific sources in the next two chapters.

In addition to the list of traits and elements, a discussion of the probable origin and cultural affiliations of each group is presented. Furthermore, the peculiar status of both Jumanos and Patarabueyes with regard to the diffusion of culture in Texas and adjacent regions and the development or modification of local cultures is discussed.

Patarabueye Traits

Bands, Tribes, Alternate Names[d]

Sixteenth Century

Patarabueyes (Tatarabueyes), Passaguates(?), Amotomancos (Otomoacos), Abriaches, Caguates, Tanpachoas(?), Cabris, People of the Cows(?).

Seventeenth Century

Julimes, Oposmes (Obomes), Polaques (Puliques), Polacmes, Conejos, Cacalotes, Mesquites, Posalmes, Conchos, Cibolas(?), Rayados(?).

Eighteenth Century

Julimes, Oposmes, Puliques, Polacmes, Conejos, Cacalotes, Mesquites, Poxalmes, Conchos, "Sibulas de San Xtobal, Puliques, and Pescados," Cocoimes, Cholomes(?), Chocolomes(?), Trigos.

Nineteenth and Twentieth Centuries

Julimenos, Pulicos, Conchos, Chalomos (Cholombos), Trigos.

Range[d,a]

Valley of the Rio Conchos from about Julimes to La Junta; valley of the Rio Grande from near Redford, south of Presidio, to a point somewhere north of Candelaria; immediately adjacent areas.

Friends and Allies[d]

Conchos, Sumas(?), Jumanos, Spaniards, and, rarely, Apaches.

Enemies[d]

Chiso bands, Apaches (usually), and Spaniards (occasionally). Others could be identified in the records.

Physical Type and Appearance

Mesocranial[a]; large stature, "handsome men and beautiful women" (Spaniards as judges), clean.[d]

Personal Adornment[d]

"Faces, arms and bodies striped with pleasing lines." Women wore hair long and tied to head; men cut hair very short over most of head but left hair of middle of head two fingers long and curled it with paint in such a way that it resembled a skull-cap. Men left scalp lock on crown of head and decorated it with black and white feathers of geese, cranes, and sparrow-hawks. "Men have their privy parts tied with a small ribbon" (Tanpachoas only).

Clothing and Jewelry

Men wore no clothing but used tanned bison hides as cloaks.[d] Women dressed in sleeveless bodice of tanned deer skin and wore another tanned deer skin as a skirt.[d] Cloaks of tanned bison skin likewise were worn by women.[d] Moccasins of bison hide, "shawls," and "ornaments like bonnets with colored feathers" or "adornments in the shape of feather caps" were noted.[d]

Jewelry, ornaments, etc., included: "a piece of copper which an Indian carried about his neck tied with some cotton threads," "... a copper sleigh bell," "white and colored coral, although not of fine quality, suspended from the nose," "turquoise."[d] Actual specimens recovered[a] include beads of *Conus, Olivella,* and other shells, shell pendants, and conch shell "bow guards"(?), long bone beads, perhaps worn in the hair, turquoise beads and polished pebbles,[a] and fragments of carved mussel shell.[a] Red pigment (hematite) molded into conical forms probably served as face and body paint.[a]

Economy

They were primarily farmers but made much use of wild plants, bison, deer, small game, and fish.[d,a] Cultivated crops included maize,[d,a] beans,[d] and calabashes (probably squash)[d,a] in the sixteenth century; wheat, maize, beans, stringbeans, watermelons, pumpkins, tobacco, and "other grains" by 1715.[d] Wild plants used included mesquite beans, mescal, prickly pear fruit, and "mushrooms."[d]

Flood irrigation apparently was employed in the sixteenth century; ditch irrigation by 1715.[d] Fish were caught with small drag nets by the Tanpachoas[d] and the presence of notched pebbles (net sinkers?) in other sites suggests that the same technique was in general use.[a] No other data available as to hunting, fishing, or collecting techniques.

Houses

Large rectangular houses built in pits

Described as "half under and half above the ground," these were joined to form long dwelling tiers. Individual houses were oriented north-south; tiers oriented east-west. House framework consisted of large posts and beams of cottonwood "the size of a man's thigh," varying in number. Support poles were placed inside house area, not along walls. Walls were made of "palings" (probably stems of the Ocatilla plant) plastered with mud and set against a pole framework. Roofs were probably flat or low-gabled, and earth-covered. Houses resembled those of the Mexicans. Several families shared same room (or at least several fires were kept going on the floor of each room). In one pueblo there were eight large houses (undoubtedly house tiers) inhabited by more than three hundred people.[1] Floors were made of tramped refuse, and no special floor features were observed. No trace of a side entrance was found but in 1715 the house faced on the plaza, which might indicate side entrances. However, the same account notes that the Spaniards stored their food "in one of the few houses of the pueblo that had doors like a presidio ...," and on several occasions the people were observed standing on the roofs of their houses, which probably but not necessarily indicates roof entrance.[d, a]

"Flat-roofed houses in their fields where they reside during harvest time"[d]

These are perhaps to be associated with circular earth lodges built in pits on a framework of four supporting posts set in the room, with inward slanting walls, brush and earth roof, and possibly pole ladders used in connection with roof entrance.[a]

Rectangular ceremonial houses(?)

These are small rectangular houses built in shallow pits with a supporting framework of two or four upright posts set in pairs inside room space, support posts at room corners in walls, and smaller vertical posts set at intervals in walls. The wall construction presumably was similar to the large rectangular houses described above, and the roofs presumably were flat. They were oriented north-south, and the north end joined to the house tier of rectangular houses. Floor was of packed earth or refuse. Rectangular plastered adobe block or "altar" set against center of south wall. Adobe-lined fire pit was built against north side of altar. This is a survival of an older secular house type.[a] The evidence for the presence of these ceremonial houses in the Concepción Focus is that of one tier of rectangular houses with two "ceremonial" structures attached, excavated at the Millington site (Shafter 7:1).

Circular ceremonial house(?)

This is a circular earth lodge similar to the circular flat-roofed house described above, but with adobe "altar" set near south side of house. One such structure was found; could not be referred unquestionably to the Concepción Focus.[a]

"Grass huts"[d]

The phrasing indicates that these were not flat-roofed houses. This may be a reference to the circular "earth lodges" described above, or it may refer to another type of house.

Storage houses

The written evidence refers to "granaries built of willow after the fashion of the Mexicans, where they keep their provisions and their harvest of mesquite and other things."[d] The corresponding archaeological structures are circular pits lined with vertical poles and grass matting(?) with floors of hard packed clay. They varied from two feet to five feet in diameter and were built near the houses.[a] The nature of the superstructure is unknown.

Villages

Documentary sources describe the following: rancherias resembling pueblos; a pueblo with a neatly kept plaza located on a high ridge; a pueblo with plaza in the middle; houses face on a plaza; a village surrounded by wall; a pueblo divided into three settlements, about 300 yards apart; and a well-built pueblo divided into two plazas, representing two united nations.[d] The archaeological evidence indicates the existence of the following: pueblos made of long east-west tiers of joined rectangular houses; isolated houses; storage houses; depressions, or large circular excavated areas, of unknown use; lodge sites, or sweat houses; midden circles; refuse heaps (Conchos Focus—mission period only); and defensive walls with boulder base (type of superstructure unknown).[a]

Population

The best estimate of the population of the La Junta pueblos is found in the census figures of Trasviña Retís in 1715. These figures purportedly represent an actual account of the populace of each pueblo, with an allowance made for those at that time working in the Conchos Valley settlements. Trasviña's figures are as follows:

Nuestra Señora de Loretto (Mesquites)	80
San Juan Bautista (Cacalotes)	165
San Francisco de La Junta (Oposmes)	180
Nuestra Señora de Aranzazu (Conejos)	71
Nuestra Señora de Guadalupe (Polacmes and Sibulas)	550
Señor San José (Puliques)	92
San Antonio de Padua (Conchos)	87
San Christóbal (Poxalmas)	180
Indians working at San Bartolomé	80
Total Population of La Junta Pueblos	1485

In addition, 44 Conejo Indians lived at Nuestra Señora de Begoña at Cuchillo Parado and 190 Cholome Indians lived farther up the Rio Conchos at San Pedro. If these are included, the total population stands at 1719 people. In 1761 Serrano spoke of 2350 people in the valley of La Junta, and noted that the population of San Juan (Bautista?) had been 400 but was reduced to half that number. Luxán estimated the population of San Francisco (Santo Tomás) at 600 Indians in 1582, and Espejo stated that there were more than 10,000 people in the valley. All accounts agree that Guadalupe pueblo was the largest of the villages, a statement in accord with the archaeological evidence.

Implements Used in War and in Obtaining Food

These included the sinew-backed bow ("Turkish, all reinforced and very strong" with strings of bison sinew) and stone-tipped arrows.[d, a] Arrow-points were small pressure-flaked points of flint. The types used were Perdiz Pointed Stem, Clinton Contracting Stem, Piedras Triple Notched, Frisco Base Notched, Saucita Split Base, and Fresno Triangular.[a] The number of specimens found indicates that hunting or warfare must have been important.

Tools customarily used in making arrows found in the La Junta sites included small slabs of sandstone, probably used in pairs to abrade the shafts; and carefully shaped stones with or without handle-like projections and having on one face a polished groove, normally used in straightening arrow shafts.[a]

Very good bison-skin shields, type unknown, were used, and "wooden bludgeons half a yard in length made of tornillo wood" were employed in fighting by the Tanpachoas.[d]

Utility Implements

Snub-nosed scrapers were probably hafted and used for scraping hides.[a] Bison hides were also prepared by "beating them with stones, until they are soft."[d] Cutting tools included double-pointed knives, ovate and triangular blades, stemmed knives, and many small flakes with chipped cutting edges.[a] Small sharp-pointed awls, with circular or ovate flake bases, nail-like drills with circular or diamond-shaped cross-section, and fine-pointed "gravers" were the characteristic piercing implements.[a]

Metates were common. They had an elongated oval bowl approaching a trough, and a backward-and-forward grinding motion seems indicated. The metates of the Conchos Focus and later were troughed specimens, lacking legs and open at both ends. Metates were placed directly on house floors, and not in bins.[a] Manos were rectangular or ovate one-hand types, ground on one or both faces. Many of them had been carefully shaped; others were river stones modified only by wear in grinding.[a] Mortars may have been used in softening bison hides, or in pounding mesquite beans.

Rare polished and grooved stone axes appear in collections, but were not found in sites. The only cutting tools of this type found were crude chipped choppers. Hard, fine-grained stones showing facets of wear probably represent stones used in polishing pottery.[a]

Pottery was made by the coiling technique, but the coils were left unmodified only on the necks of one variety. Pottery was primarily sand-tempered and the surface was smoothed, polished, or semi-polished. Red slips or washes were used. Red paint was used in pottery decoration, and striating, roughening, and punctating were texturing techniques used in decoration. Bowls, jars, and curious, heavy "trays" with low, thick side walls were made, and miniature vessels have been found. Handles or lugs were rare, and jar bottoms were predominantly pointed or sharply rounded. In the mission period (Conchos Focus) pottery was wheel-turned and sometimes partially glazed. Pottery wares include Chinati Plain, Striated, and Neck-Banded; Capote Plain and Red-on-Brown; Paloma Red-on-Gray; Conchos Plain and Red-on-Brown; and unnamed polished red wares. Pierced and unpierced pottery discs occur.[a] Pottery is not mentioned directly in the documentary sources.

Shallow rectanguloid grinding areas were cut into small boulders, probably to serve as paint mortars, and soft white tuff was carved into small bowls, often decorated on the exterior or around the rim in geometric designs.[a]

Hammerstones, rejects, and modified flint nodules occur but are not common.[a]

Gourd vessels, tanned hides, and "native blankets" were noted.[d]

Ceremonial Paraphernalia(?)

Conical "cloud-blower" stone pipes occur, but may belong only to the La Junta Focus. One fragment of the stem of a small pottery elbow-pipe of a commercial trade type(?) was found.[a]

Polished turquoise pebbles, polished stone balls or concretions with a greasy feel, and numerous odd-shaped concretions and fossils may have had ceremonial significance.[a]

A drum used in dances was described as made of "some skins attached to a vessel in the form of a tambourine."[d]

Social and Political Features

Villages were apparently autonomous units with chieftains and subchieftains. Chieftains were highly respected. A tanned bison hide was carried around to serve as a seat for the chieftain. Although there were language differences between the pueblos, intermarriage was commonplace, and the people "farmed together." A rudimentary confederacy apparently had been developed, because the cacique of the largest pueblo, in 1582, was said to be one "whom all the other caciques respected." Furthermore, references are made to the chief of all the La Junta Indians.[d]

There is some slight cause for suspecting that the villages represented patrilineal exogamous units, and may even have been totemic. The interpeter Pedro, a Patarabueye boy 13 years of age, was a native of a village near the edge of the La Junta valley near Cuchillo Parado. His "uncle," Juan Cantor, lived in the village of San Bernardino, five leagues up the Rio Grande from La Junta. Pedro's grandfather was Guaxi, chief of the

Caguate rancheria located some 44 leagues up the Rio Grande from San Bernardino. When Pedro was sent to call the people of his own rancheria down from the mountain where they had taken refuge from the Spaniards, he was asked first who he was and then who his father had been (Luxán, in Hammond and Rey 1929). These repeated references to male relatives may represent a projection of the Spanish system, but it suggests an emphasis on male relationship. The numerous references to intermarriage between the villages similarly suggest village exogamy. The possibility of some form of totemism is suggested by the village names which often refer to animals or plants: "Conejos" (rabbits), "Cacalotes" (crows), "Cibolas" (bison), "Mesquites," "Puliques," and so on. Quite probably these are simply Spanish nicknames rather than translations of Indian names, but the possibility that the alternate hypothesis holds true should be investigated. What, for example, is the meaning of "Julimes," "Passaguates" ("ayaguates" means beans in the Patarabueye tongue), "Oposmes," and "Poxalmas," if any, in neighboring Uto-Aztecan dialects? The possible interpretation of "Amotomanco" as "dwellers among the yucca plants" or some variation of that phrase has already been noted.

And if villages with single plazas represent exogamous patrilineal units, do the two plazas of Guadalupe pueblo, where two nations were said to be united for defense, represent exogamous patrilineal moieties, and perhaps even a dilute version of the Mexican *barrio* system? The same question would hold, of course, for San Francisco pueblo, which was divided into three sections some distance apart. These are tantalizing hints, but little more than that.

On somewhat safer ground, it seems plausible that the multiple hearths of the large Patarabueye rooms represent an extended family grouping, hence localized residence. Obviously, the archaeological evidence does not indicate whether this was patrilocal or matrilocal residence, and even the inference of localized residence can be challenged.

Respect for older males appears frequently in the records.[2] One other item: men, women, and children mingled freely with the Spaniards and both men and women accompanied them as they moved from village to village.

Ceremonial Features

The Spaniards were informed that the Patarabueyes had one lord, whom they called "Apalito." They pointed to the heavens and said that this lord had given them all they possessed. This probably should be regarded as a projection of Spanish beliefs, however.

Dances were performed at night. As many as three hundred Indians took part in the dance. They sat around the central fire singing and clapping their hands "with a rhythm... resembling the negroes' dances." Other music was furnished by the tambourine-like drum.

> They raise their hands toward the sun and sing a dance tune in their language, 'ayia canima' ....
>
> They do this with much compass and harmony, in such a way that though there are three hundred men in a dance, it seems as if it were being sung and danced by one only.... [Hammond and Rey 1927:21]

Espejo (Bolton 1916:175) notes that "during the three days and nights we were there they continually performed *mitotes,* balls, and dances, in their fashion, as well as after the manner of the Mexicans." Frequent reference is made to the custom of "making musical sounds with their mouths, similar to those of the flute."

Menchero, describing the Patarabueye rebellion of 1725, noted that "the Indians resolved to dance around the heads of the two fathers, and in fact had them bound up for this cruel death" (Hackett 1937:410), and describing the death of the Indian governor at a later date, states that the latter exhorted his wife and children not to "believe in the fables [of the Indians], which were all lies, and that there was but one God..." (Hackett 1937:408).[3]

Beyond these references I have been unable to find any data that can be interpreted as referring to ceremonials or to religion.[4] Notably lacking are references to shamans, priests, medicine bundles, fetishes, maize pollen, prayer sticks, and ceremonial houses.

Mortuary custom is fairly well known, although entirely from the archaeological record. Flexed inhumation beneath house floors, or in refuse, was the rule from early to late. Very few items were buried with the dead, usually only jewelry. No protective cairn was erected. There is only one instance of a departure from the normal type of inhumation. This was the burial of an old adult male beneath the floor of one of the large, circular, Pawnee-like pithouses attributed to the Concepción Focus. The burial was tightly flexed on its right side with the head to the northeast, and the face to the west. Over the head, which lay just beneath floor level, was a cairn of loose stones, among which were found two manos and a "paint mortar." The house apparently had been burned following the burial.

Relations with Other Groups

War

Patarabueye warfare sounds very much like Pueblo warfare. In their dealings with the Spaniards, we find a familiar pattern. At first, there was usually a token resistance by warriors at some distance from the village, while the village itself was deserted by all its occupants save only old men and women. Once the token resistance was overcome, usually without bloodshed, the Indians then received the Spaniards with great joy, welcoming them to their village and presenting them with food and other gifts in quantity. Later, after the priests were left on their own, rebellion would flare up and the priests would be expelled from the pueblo. Cooperation for mutual defense between the villages seems to have been better developed than among the Pueblos; this is expressed in the incipient Patarabueye confederacy. Continuing the Pueblo pattern, raids were made on occasion, usually in association with trading or hunting expeditions, but were never important nor characteristic. Patarabueye warfare thus was defensive warfare.[5]

Trade

Patarabueye trade appears to have been well developed indeed, but in a more or less passive way. That is, the Patarabueyes apparently were go-betweens rather than active, traveling traders. The aboriginal picture may be reconstructed as follows. From the west came colored feather ornaments (probably parrot feather), copper (including copper bells), coral, turquoise, cotton *mantas* in blue and white, and probably maize in quantity, at least in drought years. In exchange for these products, the Patarabueyes gave tanned hides of deer and bison. This trade was carried on with the people who adjoined them on the west, elsewhere identified as the Conchos Indians. And where did the Conchos receive these products? A Conchos Indian trader visiting the Patarabueyes told the Spaniards that 15 days' journey to the west there was a large settlement of his people, located on a very large lake, who lived in many storied houses, kept turkeys, and had maize and other provisions in quantity.[6]

This is perhaps a garbled reference to Conchos rancherias in the vicinity of Casas Grandes at this time, but they did occupy the general area. The reference to a large lake would seem to agree with this identification. As to the turkeys, maize, and other provisions in quantity, it is doubtful if this would apply to Conchos groups in northwest Chihuahua, at least at this late date. It may be suggested, however, that the Conchos were intermediaries in this trade. The Conchos are known to have been in touch with the Opata (Sauer 1934:50–61) on the northwest. The Opata themselves participated in the parrot feather-turquoise trade between southern Mexico and the Southwest (Sauer 1932:1, 2, 16–18), and their land was noted for its rich supplies of maize. From the Opata, then, the Conchos could have obtained and passed on to the Patarabueyes maize in quantity, cotton *mantas,* turquoise, parrot feathers, copper bells, and coral, intercepting the Mexican-Southwest trade in these objects, and contributing to it the prepared bison and deer skins obtained in the east.[7]

Another alternative is that the Conchos obtained the items in question from the Tepehuane or Tarahumara. In the case of the Tarahumara, at least, the trade goods in question probably were lacking, and there is no evidence of trade from either of these groups.[8]

The hides that the Patarabueyes traded to the Conchos were obtained by the former through trade with the Jumanos, and perhaps other Plains hunters as well. Undoubtedly, maize was the principal item exchanged for the hides. It is possible that the Patarabueye bows and arrows, so highly praised by the Spaniards, likewise constituted manufactured products traded eastward.[9]

So much for the aboriginal trade. In early historic times the Patarabueyes came into contact with the outlying Spanish settlements and tapped thereby a ready source of new trade goods. Metal for arrowpoints, knives, and axes, as well as jewelry, cloth, new agricultural products, and probably most important of all, horses, were the products carried eastward. In 1582 objects of iron had already reached La Junta, and by 1715 European artifacts were commonplace in the Patarabueye towns. There is no direct evidence, but it is a fair inference that the Jumanos obtained such goods in quantity at La Junta and traded them eastward.

Miscellaneous Behavior[10]

The following inferences as to Patarabueye behavior seem to be warranted and perhaps important. Nevertheless, they are inferences and accordingly should not be over emphasized.

In the records of expedition after expedition, there are references to the "merriment" with which the Spaniards were received by the Patarabueyes. In the Gallegos account of the Rodríguez expedition, for example, "[they are] very merry," "very spirited," "they showed great merriment," "they seemed to be happy," "they went away much pleased." Luxán noted that in all the pueblos the Spaniards were "received with great rejoicing." And in Trasviña's account: "[the Indians] came out to receive me with much joy"; "they gave me [presents of food] showing much joy"; "all gathered around me with rejoicing"; "they acknowledged their gratitude . . . to Colonel Masoni, because he had made their hearts happy, which is the Indian way of acknowledging their contentment. They manifested it by their actions and demonstrations." And Trasviña notes: "I found men, women, and children with good-natured, happy faces, who were very sociable with the Spaniards . . . ." Such behavior is difficult to handle in a trait list, but it seems fully as characteristic of this group as their style of hairdressing, and probably much more significant.

Furthermore, it seems clear that the Patarabueyes as a group were markedly lacking in personal aggressiveness. This characteristic is even more difficult to document. In the first place, they did not indulge to any extent in aggressive warfare. We never read of a nondefensive Patarabueye raid, either on the Spaniards or other Indians. And when their villages and fields were damaged by the encroachments of the soldiers, their reaction was to flee the pueblos, not to fight. From 1581 onward they were in contact with the Spanish settlements, but of their own accord they made no attempt, other than casual ones, to secure missions for their towns, leaving that task to be performed by the Jumanos. And I can find no reference to Patarabueye trickery, treachery, lying, or inciting of other tribes to revolt. Actually, the significance of these negative traits becomes clear only when they are placed in contrast to the Jumanos, to whom the reverse of all the statements made applies.

There is apparent in the Patarabueyes a Pueblo-like love of order and plan. The way in which the houses were fitted into a village plan, the cleanliness of the plazas, and the disciplined orderliness of village behavior all suggest this trait. But this is in part balanced by great variability in other features. Although the houses were fitted into the village plan, considerable sloppiness is evident in their construction. Houses vary slightly in size, and hence the house row is uneven and ragged. House pits were of varying depths, and probably the silhouette of the roof tops was correspondingly uneven. The house tiers did not run directly east-west but curved somewhat. Remarkably little consistency was apparent even in the fundamentals of house construction. In one house a row of small posts ran across the house floor, serving as roof supports; in another four large posts were used. In still another the posts were large but were placed in the room corners. How is such variability to be interpreted? Are we dealing with an admixture of peoples whose varying customs are only slowly being oriented in a common direction? Alternately, are we concerned with a culture whose former rigid standards are disappearing as one phase of the disintegration of the culture itself?[11] Either suggestion could be applicable in terms of known Patarabueye history, and other possibilities exist.

Affiliations and Origin of Patarabueye Culture

No attempt has been made to determine the cultural affiliations and origin of the Patarabueyes through detailed comparisons of their traits with those of other groups. Two general statements can be made with assurance: (1) Patarabueye culture is an admixture of Southwestern and Plains elements, and (2) the more recent phases were less Southwestern and more nearly Plains in affiliation.

Southwestern elements would include adobe masonry, clustered contiguous rooms, planned villages with plazas and streets, adobe block "altars," pounded adobe floors, roof entrance(?), polychrome pottery, corrugated utility pottery, neck-banded utility pottery, turquoise, woven cotton cloth, stone cloud-blower pipes, stone arrow-shaft straighteners, milling stones, flexed burials beneath house floors, semi-subterranean ceremonial rooms, pronounced directional orientation, flood irrigation, and perhaps, in a more restricted sense, a sense of order and self discipline, minimum aggressiveness, defensive warfare only. But of these, adobe masonry, pounded adobe floors, polychrome pottery, corrugated utility pottery, and perhaps cloud-blower pipes belong only to the earlier La Junta Focus.

Plains elements would include snub-nosed scrapers, double-pointed beveled knives, fine-pointed chipped awls, paired(?) sandstone shaft abraders, the type of bison and deerskin dress, hide moccasins, tanning of hides by beating them with stones(?), and perhaps pointed-bottom plain pottery, Pawnee-like arrangement of house supports in circular houses, and the sinew-backed bow, though the wider distribution of the latter items makes their inclusion here dubious.

Surprisingly, there appear to be Southeastern elements in the culture. Palisaded villages, village confederacy, great respect paid to the chief of the confederacy, special seat for the high chief, pottery with punctate decoration, and the specialized style of male hair dressing are certainly suggestive of the Southeast, especially since they occur together. On the other hand, many of these items have a wide distribution in Mexico (the same could be said of many of the putative Southwestern elements as well) and some of them occur sporadically in both the Southwest and the Plains.

Specifically Mexican items in the culture are less obvious, aside from the intrusive Mexican potsherds and copper bells. The rectangular jacale houses "look Mexican," but occur in the Southwest, and even in the Southeast. "Dances like those of the Mexicans" are noted but the meaning of the statement is uncertain.

There are some traits that are neither Southwestern nor Plains, but otherwise are of dubious provenance. Emphasis on the eating of fish, contiguous houses built in pits, and flute-like sounds made with the mouth, probably belong in this group. There are also the widespread traits: maize-beans-squash agriculture; coiled and scraped pottery; pottery decoration by texturing; earth lodges; flexed burial; and others.

Certain traits are impressively absent. The polished stone axe and maul, black-on-white pottery, the ventilator-altar-firepit-sipapu complex, stone masonry, priests, fetishes, medicine bundles, masks, temple mounds, stairways, and secondary burial are traits never recorded for the culture.

Patarabueye culture, of course, is peripheral in location to Mexico, the Southwest, the Plains, and more remotely to the Southeast. The peculiar combination of traits is approximately what one would expect, except for the weakness in specific Mexican traits and the apparent strength in Southeastern traits. The latter circumstance, I believe, results from the peculiar position and activity of the Jumanos; the former remains inexplicable. La Junta lies athwart one of the few feasible routes of travel northward from southern Mexico, and the second one discovered and followed by the Spaniards in their northward push. Why, then, was there little, if any, direct trade or movement of culture along this route during the life span of the prehistoric Patarabueye culture?

That such Mexican items (copper bells, parrot[?] feathers, potsherds) as did reach La Junta apparently came by the Opata-Conchos route is explainable in terms of historic events. Both the Chihuahua culture and the El Paso Phase can be regarded as resulting from the southward expansion of more northerly Southwestern cultures, presumably after the parrot-turquoise trade route had already come into existence. As adjacent developments they maintained trade relations even when the El Paso Phase pushed southward to La Junta and the Bravo Valley Aspect came into being. When Opata replaced the Sonora culture on the west, and Conchos replaced the Chihuahua culture, the old route was still maintained. That it was a recognized arm of the regular *camino real* northward is indicated by the fact that Ibarra in 1565 followed it as far as the vicinity of Casas Grandes (Sauer 1932:38–50).

Our knowledge of Patarabueye origins is quickly summarized. When the El Paso Phase expanded southward to La Junta, there were at least two still older cultures in possession of the land; the Chisos Focus, a modified and partially agricultural survival of the archaic hunting and collecting culture of the cave dwellers; and the Livermore Focus, a hunting culture oriented unquestionably toward the Plains. The El Paso Phase itself has been traced back to a remote Mogollon origin with Anasazi admixture.[12]

In the oldest La Junta Focus levels discovered at the Millington site (Shafter 7:1), there is a characteristic linear adobe-walled pueblo of the El Paso Phase, and close to it typical La Junta Focus pithouses. The pottery of the lowest levels is El Paso Polychrome, or else belongs to the Chihuahua series. On general arguments I suggest that a combination of the El Paso Phase with some Plains group, probably the Livermore Focus, produced the La Junta Focus.

The change from La Junta Focus to Concepción Focus could be explained as resulting from: (a) the disappearance, probably as the result of intensifying nomadic intrusion, of the Chihuahua culture and the El Paso Phase, and with them their constant reinforcement of the Southwestern elements in the Bravo Valley Aspect; (b) the intrusion into the Bravo Valley Aspect of one or more groups of Plains hunters, presumably the same nomads who brought about the changes noted above; and (c) local development. A fair argument, but not completely convincing, can be developed identifying the later Plains invaders with the pointed-bottom, plain, neck-banded, and striated-neck Chinati pottery, the large circular earth lodges, the custom of flexed burial under the house floor followed by burning of the house, and with the occupancy of one dwelling unit by several presumably related family groups. This argument can then be expanded to identify this complex as of Athapascan origin, in common with the nomadic invaders of Chihuahua. Further studies of the Bravo Valley materials, including additional excavation, will be required to prove, modify, or completely disprove this and other arguments.

The final disappearance of the Patarabueye *group* has been discussed. The disappearance of Patarabueye *culture* is another question, and one that remains to be answered. During the Conchos Focus, Spanish acculturation was completed, resulting in the breakdown of cultural and group identity. Nevertheless, *village* identities survived, and it is almost certain that there are cultural and physical survivals as well. As previously indicated, the modern house form in many instances is still quite similar to that of the Concepción Focus. The manufacture of red-on-brown pottery in familiar shapes is only now disappearing from the area (Plate II*i*). Here is fertile ground for students of acculturation and cultural survivals.

15

The Jumanos

Jumano Traits

Band, Tribes, Alternate Names[d]

Jumanos, Jumanes, Xomans, Chuman, Choman, Chouman, Chomanes, Choumanes, Choma, Human, Humanes.

Range[d,a]

Edwards Plateau, with exception of Nueces canyon region, and Trans-Pecos, with some extension into immediately adjoining regions.

Friends and Allies[d]

Patarabueyes, Cibolas of central Texas (Tonkawa?), Tejas (Hasinai), Red River Caddo(?), Tompiro of Gran Quivira(?), Iapes, Xabatoas, Jediondos, and many others. Apaches after about A.D. 1700. Friends of the Spaniards.

Enemies

Apaches, Chisos, Cuitoas, Escanjaques, Aijados, and in the eighteenth century, Comanches, Wichitas, and others.

Physical Type and Appearance[d]

Almost no data. "Most of them" said to be "flat-headed."

Personal Adornment[d]

Probably tattooed but not certain. It is a fair inference that their hair style, body painting, etc., were quite similar to that of the Patarabueyes.

Clothing and Jewelry

Said to resemble the Patarabueyes in their dress.[d] Long bird bone beads, probably worn in hair, or as tinklers on moccasin laces.[a]

Economy

Primarily traders and bison hunters.[d] Probably used shellfish, and in Trans-Pecos collected wild plants.[a] Wild plants used included mesquite, calabashes, and prickly pear. Fish may have been eaten.[1]

Agricultural products probably were obtained from Tejas and Patarabueyes through trade.[d]

Houses

Portable "tiendas"; quite probably the bison skin *tipi.* Details unknown, but there is a reference to "doors."[d]

Villages

Camps or rancherias located along streams and in rock shelters.[d,a]

Population[d]

Data variable and difficult to interpret. A rancheria near New Braunfels, Texas, was occupied by the Jumanos and five other groups. The entire assembly was said to number about 2000 Indians, or an average of over 300 persons per group. Similarly, the "Apache" rancheria located near La Junta in 1716, which may well have been a Jumano rancheria, was said to contain 60 families, hence about 300 people or less. Earlier, in 1629, the priests who visited the Jumanos on the plains found there more than 2000 persons, but other tribes than the Jumanos may have been included.

Implements Used in War and in Obtaining Food

Stone-tipped arrows,[d,a] probably used in connection with the sinew-backed bow of the Patarabueyes. Arrowpoints were small and made from flakes by the pressure technique. The actual types used included Perdiz Pointed Stem, Clifton Contracting Stem, and Fresno Triangular.[a] Arrowpoints occur in large numbers in Toyah Focus components.[a] No other weapons described.

Utility Implements

Chipped stone implements probably used in cutting, scraping, and piercing hides, and possibly in tattooing, included snub-nosed scrapers, double-pointed beveled knives, well-chipped triangular, squat triangular, and ovate blades in quantity, flake knives, sharp pointed awls with flake bases, needle-tipped "gravers," and crudely chipped hand axes.[a]

Grinding stones are not certainly associated with the Toyah Focus in central Texas, but in Trans-Pecos Texas oval-bowl metates and one-hand shaped and unshaped manos are common.[a]

Bone tools include small polished awls and eyeless needles. No data are available as to wooden implements, basketry, or other perishable materials.[a]

Pottery was used sparingly. The typical ware, Doss Redware, seems to have been coiled and scraped, and in most instances lightly polished. The paste is fine and compact, and is tempered with bone or sand. The paste color is normally brownish, the surface color yellow through brown and red. The red color usually takes the form of a light wash. Decoration of any sort is very rare; occasional sherds show simple geometric patterns crudely scratched into the fired surface. Vessel forms apparently are limited to small jars with rounded bodies, probably flat disc bases, and short, straight rims. Vessel walls are thin. Loop handles, probably in pairs, occur.[a]

A second ware, Leon Plain, is probably of Tonkawa origin rather than Jumano, but occurs in Toyah Focus components. This ware blends typologically into Doss Redware, but the distribution of the two is not identical. The surface of Leon Plain is usually poorly smoothed and bumpy, allowing the coil construction to show through. The paste is usually coarse and the tempering used is predominantly bone. Surface and paste alike range from reddish brown into dark gray in color, and the red wash of Doss Redware is missing. Again, small jars are represented, but the form is more nearly cylindrical, with narrow shoulders, long, straight rims, and somewhat pinched lips. The base is a flat, circular disc. Body walls tend to be thick. Appliqué nodes of conical shape were applied in a horizontal band extending around the rim in some specimens.[a]

Social and Political Features[d]

Jumano chieftainships were well developed, and the chief had considerable power. Typically there was one chief for several bands or groups, apparently including some non-Jumano bands united in temporary, perhaps enforced, confederacy, with subchiefs for subject bands. These "captains" issued orders to strike the tents when the time came to move to new camps. There is some evidence of the existence of a council of captains which had considerable power, delegating duties to the chieftain himself, and to others.[2]

Ceremonial Features[d]

Benavides notes: "And it was, that he [the Devil] dried up the lagoons of water... on account of which also fled the... herd[s] of buffalo... by which all these nations sustain themselves. And directly, by the medium of the Indian sorcerers, he broadcast the word that they should change their location to seek [their] food..." (Ayer 1916:59). This is probably a reference to Jumano shamans and perhaps to their control of movements of the camp. Indians were brought to the priests in great numbers to have their diseases cured; these professed to be cured after the sign of the cross was made and words of the gospel uttered over them. At least the pattern for shamanistic curing was present. The Jumanos early adopted the cross as a religious symbol from the missionaries, and in other ways professed to accept Christianity, reporting miraculous visions to the priests. On one occasion reference is made to the "customary feasts" of the Jumanos, and the Indian men and women of the Toyah Creek rancherias in 1583 performed dances between their tents "as a sign of peace." They also greeted the Spaniards with music, to celebrate their coming. The Jumano-Apaches, in association with other Apache groups in 1771, were said to have "gathered to celebrate their victory over the Comanche and Taovaya and eat some of the... prisoners whom they had captured." This is probably a reference to the ceremonial cannibalism so common in Texas and the Southeast at this time, though notably lacking in older accounts of Texas Indians.[3] In 1689 the Eagle Pass "Jumanos" erected in their camp a post on which they fastened the heads of sixteen of their enemies. Beyond these meager citations, I can find no other references to ceremonialism of any sort among the Jumanos.

Relations with Other Groups

War[d]

Jumano warfare, unlike that of the Patarabueyes, was primarily aggressive, and only incidentally defensive. On several occasions the Jumanos attempted to enlist the aid of the Spaniards in raids on the Apaches, and on other occasions we hear that warriors of various Texas tribes had joined the Jumanos in order to make war on the Spaniards. These raids appear to have been primarily for the purpose of looting and taking prisoners. On one such raid, in which the Spaniards aided the Jumanos on the Nueces River, bundles of buckskin, bison skin, and 200 prisoners were taken. A secondary type of warfare, and one which became increasingly important as the Apaches moved southward, was that caused by the struggle for possession of the bison herds and hunting territory. Jumano warfare probably falls into the Plains pattern, although no data are available regarding scalping, counting coup, or prestige based on bravery and daring.

Trade[d,a]

The Jumanos were aggressive traders of the highest order. Bison hides and buckskin were the basic products which they obtained in the bison plains. Meat, salt, perhaps *bois d'arc* or Osage orange wood for bows, and slaves probably were traded (Swanton 1942:188–89). Bows and arrows may have been traded eastward from the La Junta towns or southwestward from the Tejas towns to the peoples of the Coastal Plain and the Gulf Coast itself, and may in fact represent one of the first items of trade used in dealing with the coastal tribes. Certainly, when the Karankawa of the Rockport Focus first began using stone-tipped arrows they adopted the type Perdiz Pointed Stem, used both by the Jumanos of the Toyah Focus, and the Patarabueyes of the Bravo Valley Aspect. Since this type was likewise characteristic of the Frankston Focus of the Hasinai, the arrows may have been obtained from that source. But even the Hasinai probably obtained this type from the Jumanos and ultimately from the Patarabueyes, inasmuch as the type is much older in the Bravo Valley Aspect than elsewhere in Texas. It may be suggested that the sinew-backed bow, if not the bow itself, was introduced into central and southern Texas, perhaps even into parts of eastern Texas, by just this trade (Fig. 14). Before the appearance of the Toyah Focus in this region, arrowpoints are unknown in the archaeological sites, and in several instances the type of arrowpoint first adopted was the Perdiz Pointed Stem, or some variation of this type. We learn from Cabeza de Vaca that the bow and arrow was widespread in south Texas in the early sixteenth century, but a close examination of his statements indicates that most of the bows and arrows were still obtained through trade,[4] and that the weapon had not yet been fully integrated into the aboriginal culture of the area. This provides us with a chronological landmark for the introduction of the bow and arrow, or at least the bow (possibly the sinew-backed bow) and stone-tipped arrows.[5] On this evidence a date near A.D. 1500 for the appearance of the stone-tipped arrow, the beginning of cultures such as the Rockport and Nueces foci, and the appearance of the Toyah Focus in south-central Texas seems reasonable (Fig. 14). An important inference to be drawn from this is that the beginning of Jumano trade in central Texas, with all that it signifies, took place on a prehistoric and pre-horse transport level.

The Jumanos were strategically located for success in such trade. Hides obtained in central Texas could be traded either westward to the Patarabueyes, and thus introduced into the Southwestern and northern

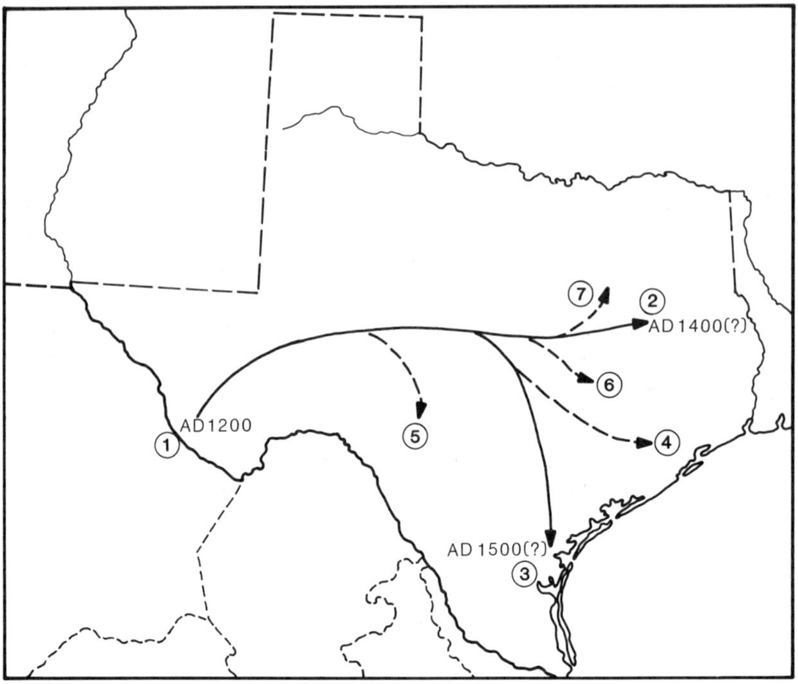

Figure 14. Hypothetical diffusion of Perdiz Pointed Stem.

Mexican stream of trade, or eastward to the Hasinai and the Southeastern trade channels. Maize could be obtained in exchange in either area. In the east, furthermore, the wood of the Osage orange could be obtained and carried westward. In the west, from the Patarabueyes, could be obtained turquoise, cotton cloth, copper bells, perhaps sinew-backed bows, arrows, and other articles for trade either to the south and central Texas tribes or eastward to the Hasinai.[6] Pottery could be obtained in either the east or west, or from the Pueblos in New Mexico. From the south by either direct or indirect barter, in exchange for maize, hides, flint, and manufactured items such as bows and arrows, could be obtained shells and other coastal products.

After the Patarabueyes on the west came into close contact with the Spaniards of Santa Barbara and Parral, that is, after about 1563, horses and other European products were introduced into this native system of trade. As already indicated, horses, items of metal, cloth, and other items reached the Hasinai before they were visited by La Salle's party in the 1680s but after the visit of the De Soto expedition in 1542. In the time of Juan Sabeata, this trade must have been at its height, accounting in part for the notoriety of the Jumanos.[7]

Archaeological evidence verifies the historical accounts. At La Junta, dating to an early historic or late prehistoric horizon, pottery of Hasinai origin was found. Here also were found occasional arrowpoints of types used in the early historic Allen Focus of the Hasinai. As already noted, Hasinai pottery likewise occurs in the Toyah-Austin foci sites along the Colorado River. And in the Allen Focus sites of the Hasinai, rare examples occur of the arrowpoint type Saucita Split Base of the Bravo Valley Aspect, together with a local "copy" of it, and numerous objects of European origin.

There is another aspect to this widespread Jumano system of trade that is of special anthropological interest. At Parral, in 1689, Juan Sabeata attributed his delay in coming to La Junta, in part, to his habit of making side trips to the various rancherias to collect news. The Jumanos, by Sabeata's own statement in 1683, at that time maintained friendly relations and carried on barter and exchange with over 36 Indian nations, including such distant tribes as the Quiviras (Wichitas), the Patarabueyes, and the Tejas (Hackett 1931:138–39).[8] Sabeata not only collected the news, he passed it on as well. It was through the accounts of the Jumanos that the Spaniards in New Mexico first heard of the Tejas. In El Paso, in 1683, Sabeata passed on to the Spaniards a bit of news collected from the Tejas themselves: "These have told this declarant that into that eastern region Spaniards [Europeans] are entering by water in wooden houses, and that they barter and exchange with the said nation of the Tejas" (Hackett 1931:139). This is prior to the establishment of the French fort on the Garcitas River and perhaps refers to La Salle's descent of the Mississippi in 1681. For additional examples of the detail with which news was conveyed by the Jumanos, review the accounts they gave the French of the Spaniards and the Spaniards of the French. The extent to which such news-bearing could go is indicated by the reports given the Spaniards in Coahuila regarding the Tejas located over 500 miles away.

> Coahuila has as a neighbor on the north, inclining somewhat to the east, a populous nation of people, and so extensive that those who give detailed reports of them do not know where it ends. These [who give the reports] are many, through having communicated with the people of that nation, which they call Texas, and who, they maintain, live under an organized government, congregated in their pueblos, and governed by a casique [*sic*] who is named by the Great Lord, as they call the one who rules them all, and who, they say, resides in the interior. They have houses made of wood, cultivate the soil, plant maize and other crops, wear clothes, and punish misdemeanors, especially theft. [Bolton 1912:16]

Apparently, a detailed knowledge of the behavior of peoples located even at great distances was circulated through the medium of just such gossip. If the Indians of Coahuila had such detailed knowledge of the Tejas in 1676, one wonders how detailed a knowledge the early Southeastern peoples had of Huastecan culture in A.D. 500, and how many of the Huastecan traits they adopted—and adapted almost beyond recognition—as a result of this knowledge. Such diffusion, even when actual objects were carried, would leave little trace and would probably result in just such vague similarities as those that puzzle the student of Southeast-Mexican relationships. This entire topic requires close scrutiny not only by students of American culture history, but by those who regard themselves as specialists in diffusion studies as well.

A word should be said about the "fairs," noted on several occasions in previous pages, which the Jumanos attended in central or south Texas. This phrasing may simply have referred to their customary bartering with the Texas tribes, but it sounds as if a more specialized sort of trade relationship, or actual market, is indicated. It will be recalled that the Indians who brought bows to the tribes of the coastal plain did so in the fall of every year at the time of the prickly pear harvest in the great thickets on the coastal plain southwest of San Antonio. This was in general a time of ample food and great feasting when Indians of many different nations and languages came together in relative friendship for a few short weeks. This would have been an ideal occasion for the exchange of goods and news, and may well represent the "fairs" in which the Jumanos participated.

Miscellaneous Behavior[d]

Just as the Patarabueyes were characterized as nonaggressive in their relationships, the Jumanos can be identified by their extremely aggressive behavior. The nature and extent of their trading expeditions, their long journeys made for the purpose of bringing the Spaniards into their land, the type of warfare practiced, are merely expressions of this clearly apparent general orientation. Furthermore, the Jumanos were constantly embroiled in intrigue, in urging the Spaniards to fight the French, or vice versa, or in persuading the Spaniards that the Apaches were about to attack them so that they would attack the Apaches. They made up highly imaginative stories to support their claims. Almost invariably the Spaniards with whom they were associated came to distrust them and regard them as thieves and liars. In the Jumanos we are dealing with an aggressive, political-minded, and commercial-minded group, contrasting greatly with the Patarabueyes, with whom they have so often been confused.

Affiliations and Origin of Jumano Culture

Such fragmentary data as we possess regarding Jumano culture and behavior point conclusively to a Plains orientation: an economy based on bison hunting, raiding, and trading; nomadic existence both with and without the aid of the horse; the use of the tipi and apparently Plains-style skin clothing; the Plains stone complex, which includes the snub-nosed scraper, double-pointed stone knife and graver; and various other items and characteristics. In spite of their close association with the Patarabueyes, I am unable to identify traits of Southwestern origin in their culture; the same applies to Mexico, and, with the possible exception of style of hair dress, to the Southeast as well.

There is little information as to the origin of the Jumanos. They may have been Patarabueyes who left their Rio Grande villages and sedentary existence to lead a life of hunting, raiding, and trading on the plains, but this seems unlikely, as the differences between the groups are so great. I believe that the Jumanos must be regarded as survivors of some Plains tribe that pushed into the Trans-Pecos and there developed the Toyah Focus. They may have been descendants of the peoples of the earlier Livermore Focus, who were likewise invaders from the Plains, or they may represent a later intrusion from that area, perhaps of Athapascan affiliation. If the latter possibility is upheld, the invaders may have introduced into Patarabueye culture those traits that changed the La Junta Focus into the Concepción Focus. As to their relations at La Junta, it seems to me clear that the Jumanos were merely tangential participants, at best, in the Patarabueye confederacy, and perhaps no more than perennial visiting traders. Their disappearance as a group seems accounted for by their absorption into the Apaches.

General Conclusions

Practically all specific conclusions of importance have been summarized in the preceding pages. Only a few general statements are needed to bring this discussion to a close.

I believe that the evidence amply substantiates the existence of a separate Jumano tribe. The Jumanos and the Patarabueyes were clearly distinct groups. Their relationship at La Junta seems to me to be comparable to that which existed between Pueblo farmer and Plains hunter at Pecos pueblo in New Mexico.

The mingling of diverse ethnic and linguistic groups living in separate pueblos and yet sharing a common culture at La Junta itself recalls the situation in the Rio Grande much farther to the north. But the people of the upper river were Puebloans who were exposed but little to any other influences save that of Plains culture, while those of La Junta brought with them into the area a mixed cultural heritage which was further diversified by a barrage of new traits from both the Southeast and Plains, and, to a much lesser extent, from Mexico.

The Patarabueyes and the Jumanos were links in a great aboriginal trade network which was certainly responsible for the exchange of not only trade commodities, but of ideas as well, between widely separated peoples of diverse cultural affiliation. This trade network probably expedited the exchange of goods and ideas between the Southwest and the Southeast, and perhaps even between Mexico and the Southwest, the Plains, and the Southeast. I regard this particular trade network as of too recent origin, however, to have contributed greatly to the development of either Southwestern or Southeastern culture. Nevertheless, late modifications may have resulted in any of these areas from ideas and artifacts exchanged through this medium. In particular, careful study is needed of the origin and diffusion of such items as the Plains headdress, peyote, neck-banded pottery in the Southeast, and the custom of torture of captives on a vertical frame, with due regard to the phenomena discussed in this paper.

The concept of stimulus diffusion, and especially that phase concerned with the movement of ideas across great distances and through cultures which remain unaffected thereby to result in modification of distant cultures, requires thorough investigation. The instance of the movement of "news" across Texas in just such a way by peoples like the Jumanos suggests that the process may have been of some significance in American culture history.

Finally, the combination of archaeological and ethnohistorical methods in attacking a specific problem has proven itself of sufficient value to suggest the utility of such studies, particularly as a future approach to problems of general anthropological theory, such as the concept of stimulus diffusion referred to above. This is not a new approach, of course, but it is one which could be applied effectively in many more instances and in a more intensified manner than is now the case.

Plates

Plate I. The Bravo Valley Aspect. *A.* Modern jacale, similar to house type of the Concepción Focus. Village of La Junta, near Loma Alta site. *B.* Excavations in progress in House Group I, Concepción Focus, Loma Alta site. Valley of La Junta in background. *C.* An excavated house of the La Junta Focus, Millington site.

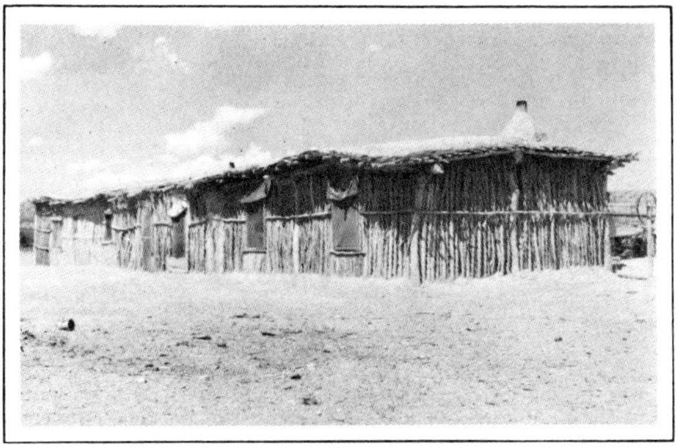

A

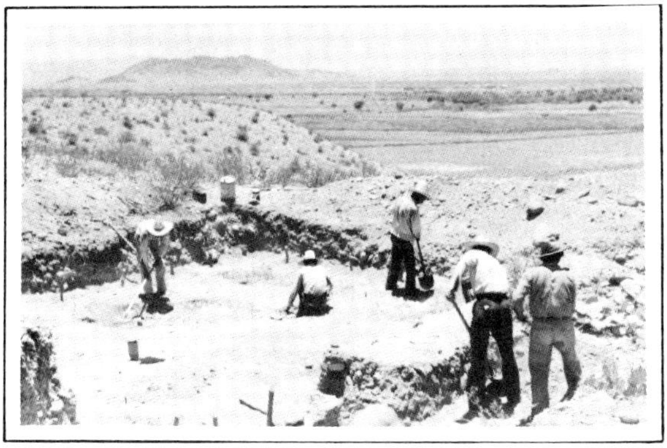

B

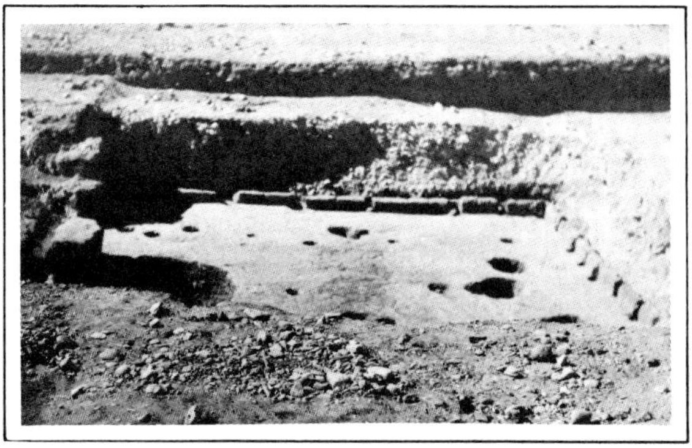

C

Plate II. Pottery of the Bravo Valley Aspect. *a.* Restored jar of Chinati Plain, Loma Alta site (max. width 22 cm). *b.* Chinati Striated-Neck. *c.* Chinati Neck-Banded. *d.* Rare sherd of Chinati Punctate-Incised. *e.* Unnamed polished redware of the Concepción Focus. *f.* Paloma Red-on-Gray (Concepción Focus). *g.* Capote Red-on-Brown (Early Conchos Focus). *h.* Conchos Red-on-Brown (Conchos Focus). *i.* Modern variant of Conchos Red-on-Brown (max. width 27 cm). *j-v.* Intrusive types (trade ware?). *j.* Restored olla of El Paso Polychrome, La Junta Focus, Shafter 7:1 (max. width ca. 60 cm). *k.* Ramos Polychrome, La Junta Focus. *l.* Villa Ahumada Polychrome, La Junta Focus. *m.* Unidentified black-on-gray (probably a duochrome related to the Chihuahua series), La Junta Focus. *n.* Chupadero Black-on-White, La Junta Focus. *o.* Majolica ware (Spanish glazed ware), Early Conchos Focus. *p.* "Colonial" or "Late Aztec" ware, La Junta Focus. *q.* "Plumbate" ware. *r.* Polished black-on-red ware (Madera Black-on-Red or Aztec ware?), La Junta Focus. *s.* Polished black-on-red ware (affinis Aztec or Madera Black-on-Red?), La Junta Focus. *t.* Polished black-on-red ware (Madera Black-on-Red?), Concepción Focus. *u.* Sherds of Patton Engraved from Concepción Focus, Shafter 7:1. Compare with whole vessel of Patten Engraved from a component of the Allen Focus in east Texas, shown at *v.* (max. width 23 cm).

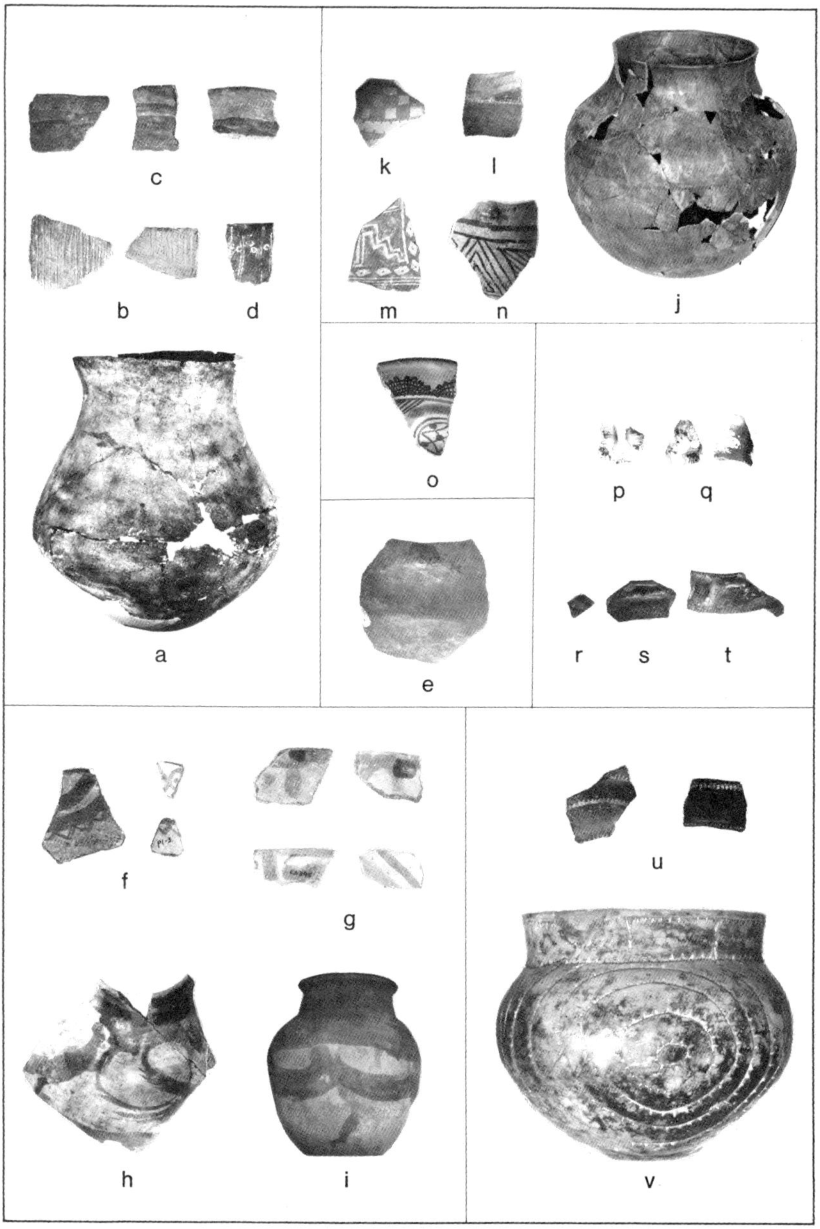
c
b
d
k
l
m
n
j
a
o
p
q
e
r
s
t
f
g
u
h
i
v

Plate III. Artifacts of the Bravo Valley Aspect. *A*. Artifacts of shell and bone. *B*. Arrowpoints and gravers. *C*. Miscellaneous chipped stone artifacts, including drills, stemmed knives, flake knives, and snub-nosed scrapers. *D*. Objects of metal, Concepción Focus and modern.

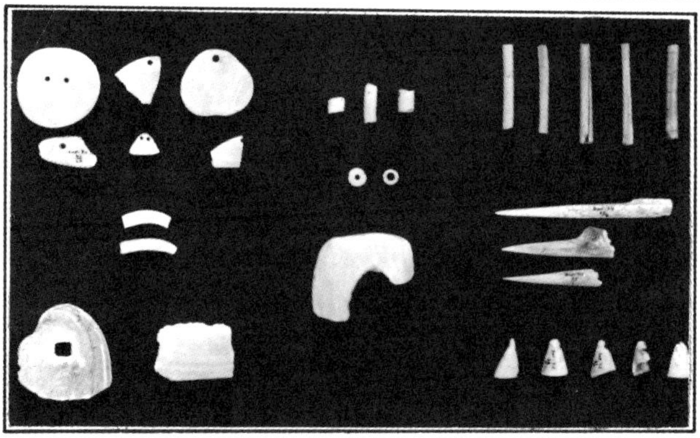

A

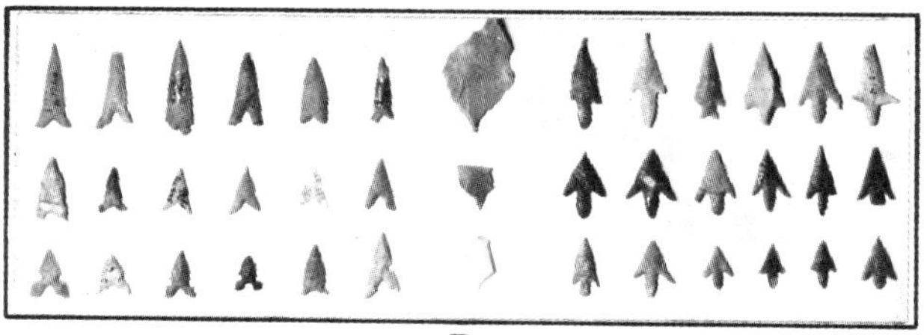

B

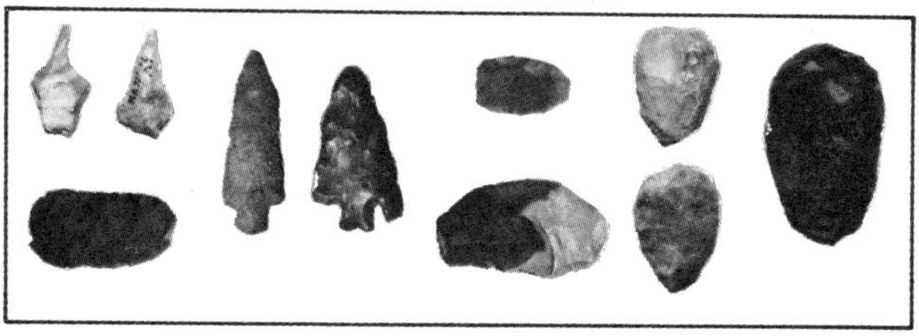

C

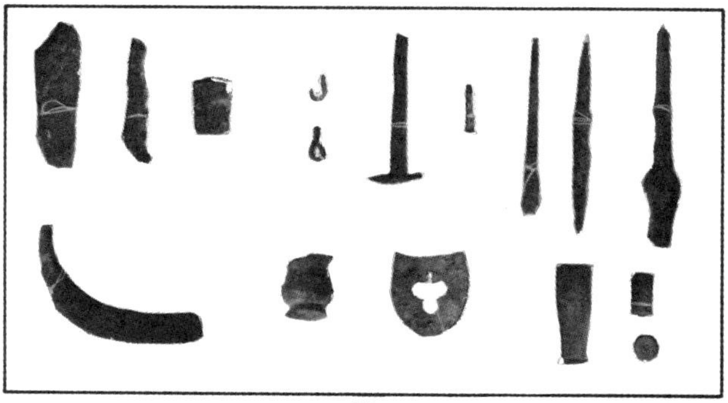

D

Plate IV. Miscellaneous artifacts of the Bravo Valley Aspect. *a.* Ground stone pipes, or "cloud blowers." *b.* Chipped hand axe (small). *c.* Fragment of carved stone bowl (volcanic tuff). *d.* Characteristic arrowshaft tools. *e.* Simple arrow-shaft tool. *f.* Arrow-shaft abrader (sandstone). *g.* Pebbles, notched at ends, and showing wear longitudinally between notches (netsinkers?). *h.* Paint mortar? *i.* Trough metate, Conchos Focus and modern. *j.* Characteristic slab metate with oval area of wear forming bowl. *k.* Mano, unshaped. *l.* Mano, shaped. *m.* Mortar. *n.* Pestle.

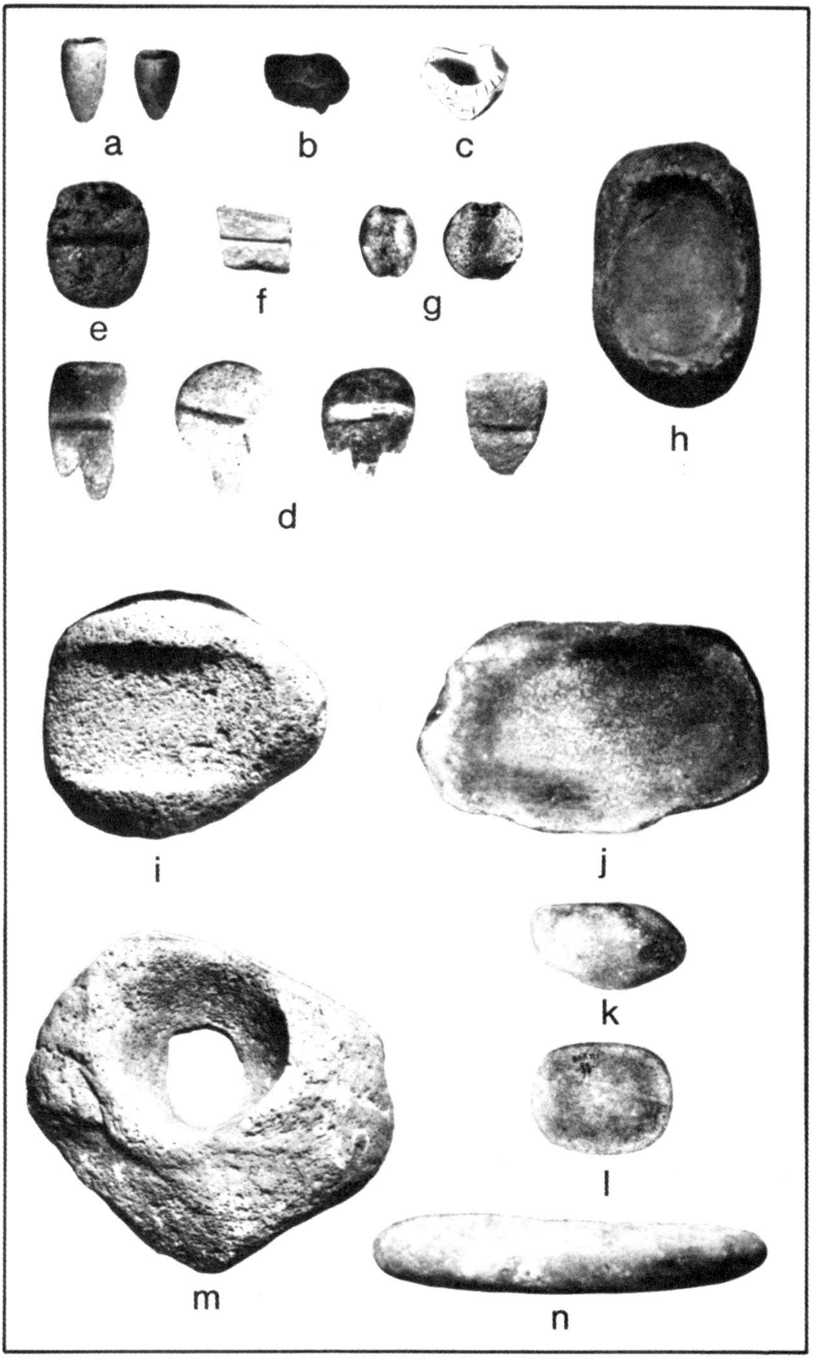
a
b
c
e
f
g
h
d
i
j
k
l
m
n

Plate V. The Lehmann rockshelter. *A*. General view of shelter. *B*. Interior of shelter, showing deposits, rear wall (covered with pictographs, not visible here), and fallen "table rocks" (right). *C*. Pictographs on rear wall of shelter. *D*. Flexed burial attributed to the Toyah Focus. Surrounding stone slabs have been removed. A bone bead is visible on foot.

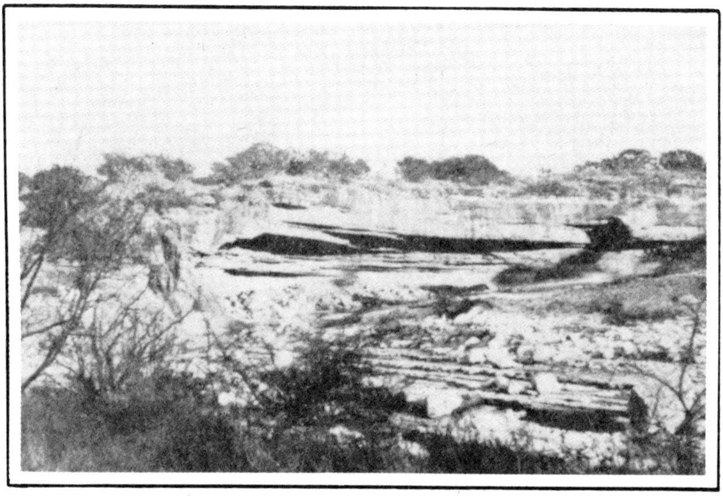

A

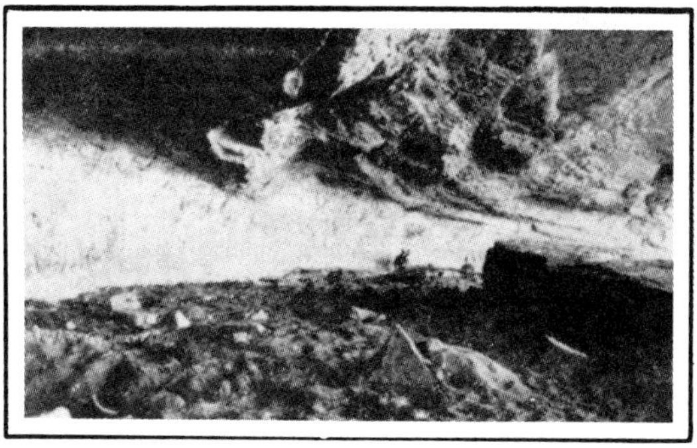

B

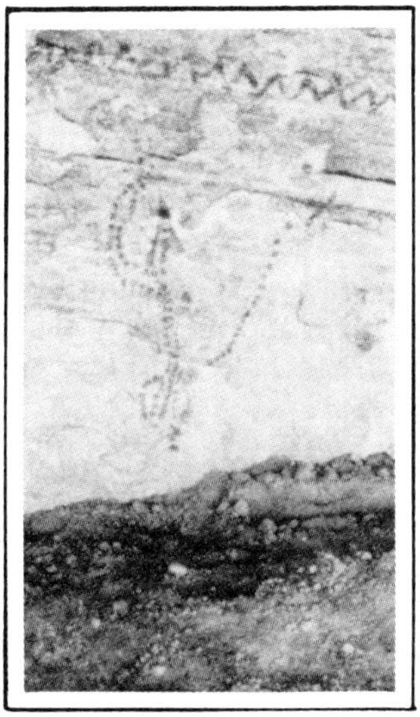

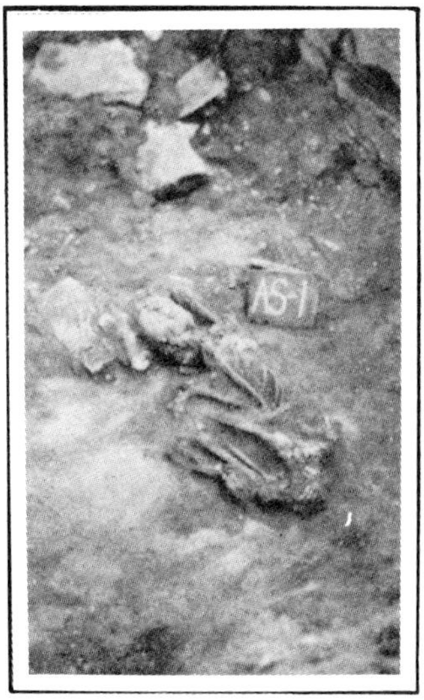

C

D

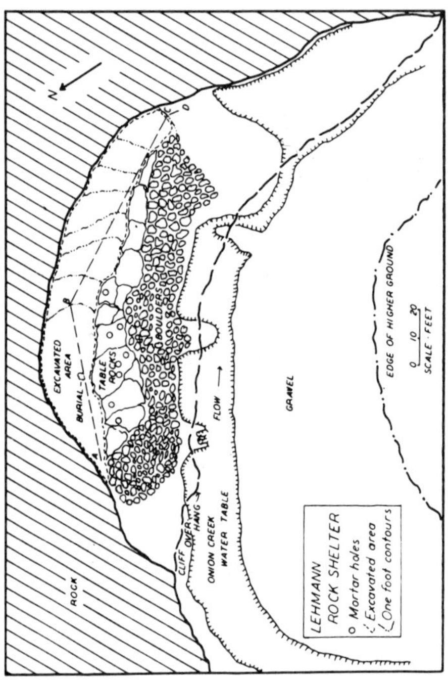
LEHMANN
ROCK SHELTER
Mortar holes
Excavated area
One foot contours
ROCK
EXCAVATED AREA
BURIAL
TABLE ROCKS
BOULDERS
CLIFF OVERHANG
ONION CREEK
WATER TABLE
FLOW
GRAVEL
EDGE OF HIGHER GROUND
0 10 20
SCALE · FEET
N

A

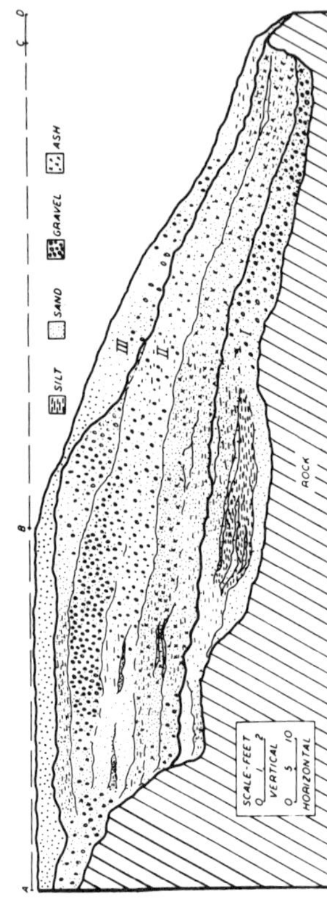
SILT
SAND
GRAVEL
ASH
ROCK
SCALE · FEET
0 1 2
VERTICAL
0 5 10
HORIZONTAL

B

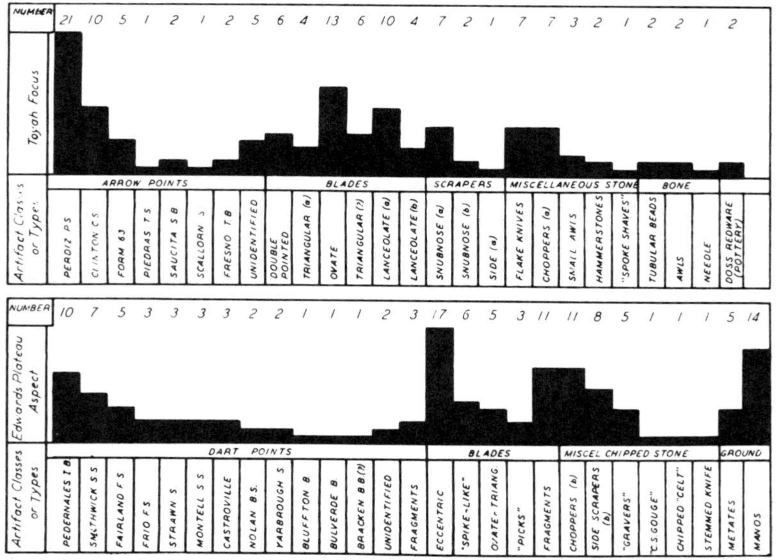

C

Plate VI. Plan, profile of deposits, and cultural composition of the Lehmann rockshelter. *A*. Plan. *B*. Composite stratigraphy. *C*. Cultural composition of Toyah Focus and Edwards Plateau Aspect components.

Plate VII. Artifacts attributed to the Toyah Focus component in the Lehmann rockshelter. *a.* Perdiz Pointed Stem point. *b.* Clinton Contracting Stem point. *c.* "Form 63" (probably Eddy Expanding Stem point). *d.* Piedras Triple-Notched point. *e.* Saucita Split Base point. *f.* Scallorn Stemmed point. *g.* Fresno Triangular Blade point. *h.* Unnamed arrowpoint type. *i.* Dulce Stemmed point. *j-l.* Snub-nosed scrapers. *m.* Small drill with flake base. *n.* Bone tube or bead. *o.* Flake sidescraper. *p-q, s-u.* Well-chipped blade. *r.* Double-pointed beveled knife.

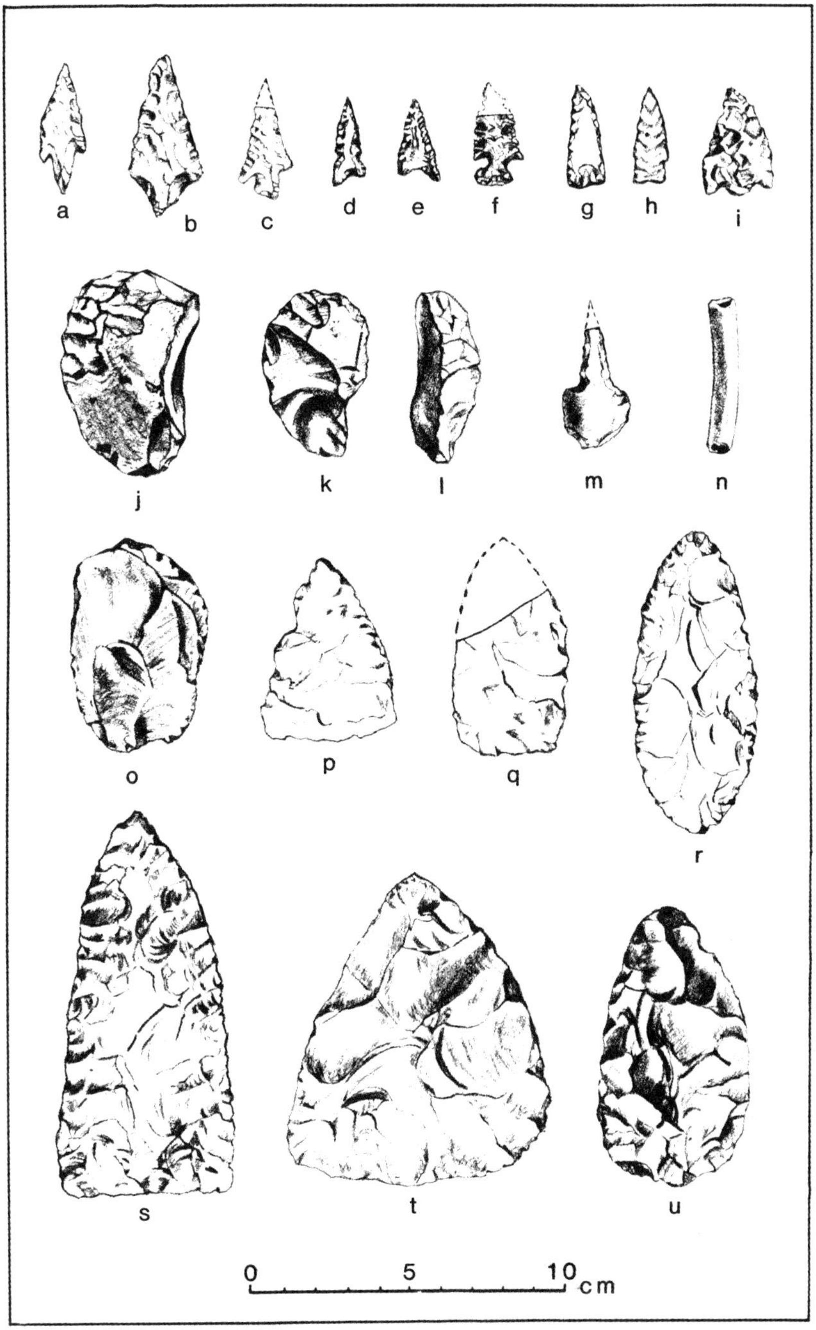
a
b
c
d
e
f
g
h
i
j
k
l
m
n
o
p
q
r
s
t
u
0
5
10
cm

Plate VIII. Artifacts attributed to the Edwards Plateau Aspect component in the Lehmann rockshelter. *a.* Pedernales Indented Base point. *b.* Smithwick Small Stem point. *c.* Fairland Flared Stem point. *d.* Frio Flared Stem point. *e.* Strawn Stemmed point. *f.* Montell Split Base point. *g.* Nolan Beveled Stem point. *h.* Yarbrough Stemmed point. *i.* Bluffton Barbed point. *j.* Bulverde Barbed point. *k.* Spike-like blade. *l-m.* Clear Fork gouge. *n.* Small triangular blade. *o.* Heavy pick-like blade. *p-q.* Heavy flake sidescraper. *r.* "Chipped celt." *s.* Percussion-chipped chopper. *t.* One-hand unshaped mano.

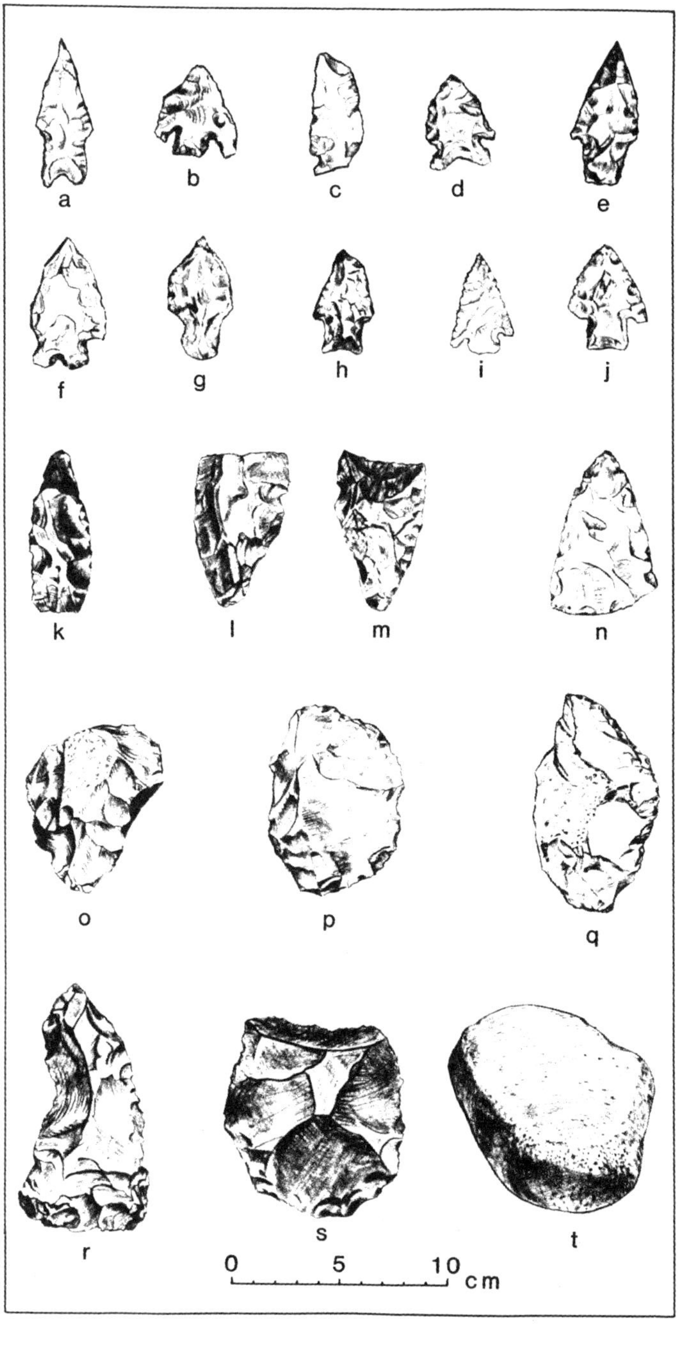
a
b
c
d
e
f
g
h
i
j
k
l
m
n
o
p
q
r
s
t
0 5 10 cm

Plate IX. Artifacts of miscellaneous Texas cultures. *a.* Toyah Focus artifacts from the Trans-Pecos region (*top,* snub-nosed scrapers; *middle,* Perdiz Pointed Stem points and one Saucita Split Base point; *bottom,* brown pottery). *b.* Doss Redware from Toyah Focus components in central Texas. *c.* Eddy Expanding Stem points (Nueces and Austin foci). *d.* Steiner Serrate points (Trading House Focus). *e.* Diminutive Frio Flared Stem points (Nueces Focus). *f.* Scallorn Stemmed and Eddy Expanding Stem (*right*) points (Austin Focus). *g.* Miscellaneous unsorted arrowpoints and other artifacts of the Livermore Focus.

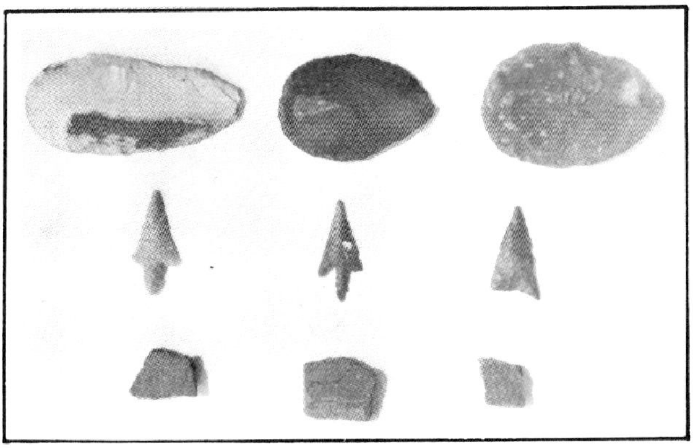

a

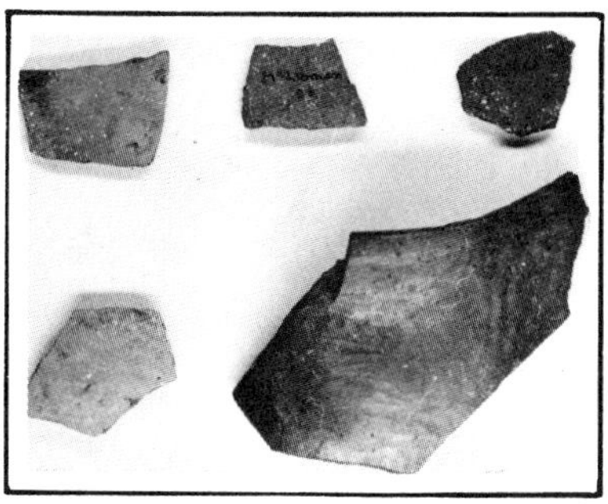

b

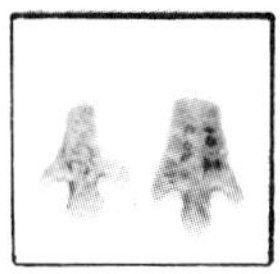

c

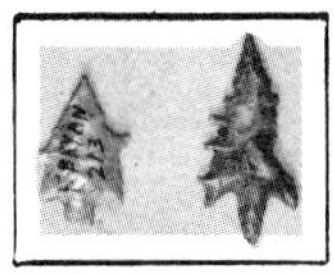

d

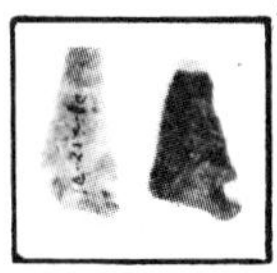

e

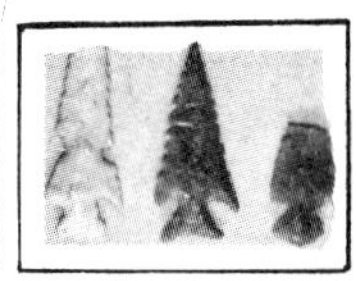

f

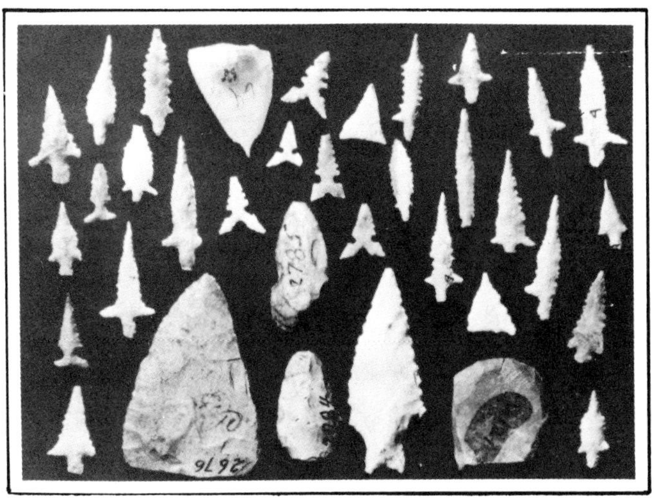

g

Notes

Introduction

1. Pichardo, in Hackett 1931:137–39, 1934:169–70, 424–27.

Chapter 2

1. This is according to Bolton's (1916) translation, which reads: "who call themselves Jumanos." Scholes pointed out that it might be more accurately translated: "who are called Jumanos." Scholes notes, however, that Obregón had interpreted the phrase as Bolton later did (Scholes 1940:275n.).
2. Luxán, in Hammond and Rey 1929:124. "We met three Jumanas Indians who were hunting and we were able to understand them through Pedro, a Pataraguey Indian belonging to Diego Pérez de Luxán. They said that the Rio de las Bacas [Pecos] came out very far down from the Conchos river; that they would take us by good roads to the junction of the Rio del Norte and Conchos river, which is among the Pataragueyes." For data regarding the location of the Jumano rancherias on Toyah Creek, see Kelley 1937:9–10, 15–16.
3. Luxán, in Hammond and Rey 1929:124–25. The Spanish text (copied from Hammond's transcription, which he loaned me) reads: "rancheada gente de esta nacion que es en el traje de manera eseto en las casas como los pataragueyes."
4. De Vaca, in Hodge 1907:104–5, and in Bandelier 1905:157. Hodge translates it "pipkins" rather than pots, but the implication is the same.

Chapter 3

1. See Oñate, "Account of the Journey to the Salines, the Xumanas, and the Sea, 1599," in Bolton 1916:234. This is a translation of a longer manuscript entitled "Relaciones que envió Don Juan de Oñate de algunas jornadas" in the Lowery Collection, Library of Congress.
2. Oñate, "Account of the Discovery of the Buffalo, 1599," in Bolton 1916. See page 225: "They asked him for aid against the Xumanas, as they call a tribe of Indians who are painted after the manner of the Chichimecos."

Chapter 4

1. "An Historical Journey of the Late Monsieur de La Salle's Last Voyage to North America...," in Stiles 1906:126. For the location of the La Salle fort, see Bolton 1924.
2. Joutel, in Stiles 1906:28–29. Also see "Narrative of La Salle's attempt to Ascend the Mississippi in 1687," in Cox 1905:241.
3. The name of the Cibola chief is given as Don Nicolás in the first testimony; later it becomes clear that only one Don Nicolás is concerned, and he is the Julimes governor from La Junta, while the chief who had sent word of his coming was actually Juan Sabeata.
4. That is, Miguel was captain of the Jumanos and Cibolas who lived at La Junta; Sabeata was governor of all the Cibolas and Jumanos. This is a clear indication that only a part, at most, of the Jumano-Cibola group lived the year around at La Junta. Instead of the Rio Grande, the river here referred to may have been the Colorado.
5. *Rescates* is the term used. This is defined as "ransom; redemption; ransom money; exchange, barter," in Appleton's New Spanish Dictionary.
6. In all probability, the "upper Rio del Norte" is actually the upper Colorado river. The river on which the Jumanos and Cibolas in central Texas had their rancherias appears to have been the lower or middle part of the Colorado, which emptied into "Espiritu Santo" Bay (Matagorda Bay). At this time the Spaniards were under the impression that the Rio del Norte was the river that flowed into Espiritu Santo Bay; hence, they interpreted Indian references to the Colorado as referring to the "Rio del Norte" (see letter of "Don Juan Isidro de Pardiñas... to His Majesty, 1688," in Hackett 1926:233). The "nations of the upper Rio del Norte" therefore probably were the Indians of the Concho River, and other upper branches of the Colorado, where the Jumanos often were found. The two rivers are confused throughout the testimony.
7. The "frigate painted on a parchment with some written annotations" survives in the archives and is illustrated in Hackett 1926.
8. This is implicit throughout the testimony of Don Nicolás and Juan de Salaises, although it is nowhere stated in so many words. On the other hand, in the testimony of Juan Sabeata in Parral in July, 1692 ("Auto," in Hackett 1926:285–89), there is an apparently contradictory statement: "[Sabeata] went to the pueblo of San Antonio [de Julimes, on the Rio Conchos of Chihuahua, above Cuchillo Parado] in search of the governor of the Julimes, in order to ask him to go to La Junta de los Ríos and aid him with four or five hundred of his own Indians against the said [enemy] nations..."
9. This is not too clear. Sabeata states "that through some Indians who have come to their rancherias [the Jumano rancherias] from this camp [Parral] and from the labor on its hacienda, they have learned of the good opinion that the natives have of the... governor" (Hackett 1926:261). This probably refers to the Julimes, who were in constant contact with the Jumanos at La Junta and the Spaniards at Parral, but other interpretations are possible. However, Fray Colina spoke of "the departure of the poor Indians to work on the haciendas."
10. "The Cibolos [and Jumanos], who come from the direction of the east to trade and bargain with [the Julimes] as friends, as they are..." From "Declaration of Juan Salaises," in Hackett 1926:237. See also "Declaration of Fray Agustín de Colina" (Hackett 1926:241–42), and "Declaration of Miguel, Captain of the Cibolos" (Hackett 1926:269–73).
11. This is by no means certain, however. When Retana reached La Junta, he took Jumanos and Cibolas as his guides; at least he took Indians who were subject to the rule of Sabeata, who was chief of the Jumanos and Cibolas. At that time Sabeata and his party were still east of La Junta, returning from central Texas, indicating that not all of his subjects had accompanied him. It is possible, however, that the the Indians whom Retana used for guides were the messengers that Sabeata had sent in advance to announce his coming.

12. For a possible identification of these Cibolas with the historic Tonkawa Indians, see Chapter 11.
13. See "Declaration of Another Heathen Indian," in Hackett 1926:281: "in order to go to Río de las Nueces..."
14. See "Declaration of the Governor of the Cíbolas," and "Declaration of a Heathen Indian," in Hackett 1926:263–69, 273–77.
15. "[T]hey made side trips to the different rancherias of Indians to collect news...," from "Declaration of Miguel," in Hackett 1926:273.
16. The references are worth repeating here:

    > they would have come earlier but for the fact that the time for going into the interior to the fairs which they conduct with the nations of the upper Río del Norte [here, the Colorado River], the Texas, and many other Indian nations, prevented them from doing so .... ["The Governor arrives...," in Hackett 1926:261]

    Sabeata continues,

    > and because it was time to go to their fairs with the Texas Indians and other nations that live along those rivers, he resolved to enter, as they did, according to custom...
    >
    > with those in his company he says that he went on nearly to the sea and was at the fairs held with the nations of Indians who live there. ["Declaration of the Governor...," in Hackett 1926:265]

    Miguel noted that

    > then the declarant and Don Juan Xaviata... were appointed to go at the time of their fairs to where the said strangers were. When the time came they proceeded by way of the lower Rio del Norte .... ["Declaration of Miguel...," in Hackett 1926:271]

    Cuis Benive stated that

    > they resolved to go to the fairs with the other nations and to find out where those people were living

    and

    > when they go to the fairs they are delayed a long time by the cold and its rigors; accordingly they set out to go to them when the trees begin to sprout, and return when the leaves are falling. ["Declaration of a Heathen Indian," in Hackett 1926:274–77]

17. "Declaration of the Governor...," and "Declaration of Miguel...," in Hackett 1926:263–73. See Chapter 5 regarding the disappearance of the Frenchman.
18. Massanet uses "Choma," and Teran, "Jumana," but both terms refer to the Indians led by Juan Sabeata.
19. "Itinerary and Daily Account Kept by General Domingo de Teran...," in Hatcher 1932:15.
20. "Diary Kept by the Missionaries...," in Hatcher 1932:57–58.
21. Bolton 1911:78–79, citing "Dictamen Fiscal" in Memoria de Nueva España, XXVII, 185. I have not been able to examine this document. For discussion of the Eagle Pass division of the Jumanos, see Chapter 5.

Chapter 5

1. Alonso de León, "Auto de los Suscido en la Jornada," in Portillo 1886:221–24.
2. "Declaración del Indio Diego de León," in Portillo 1886:237–38.
3. The repeated use of this variant form "Chome" in the Eagle Pass vicinity may be significant. "Choma" is a frequent variant applied to Sabeata's followers, but the use of "Chome" is not certain.
4. "Diary Kept by the Missionaries," in Hatcher 1932:50.

Chapter 6

1. The original documents, translated in Bolton 1911:79–84, include "Letter of July 4, 1733" (Archivo General y Público de Mexico); "Diferentes Noticias de Indios de

como ay Españoles azia los Texas" (Archivo General y Público de Mexico); "Representación" (Memoria de Nueva Espana, XXVII, 160); "Declaración del Indio Gerónimo" (1724 manuscript); "Alaman to the Viceroy, 1731" (Bexar Archives); "Testimony of Antonio de los Santos, August 21, 1734" (Bexar Archives); "Memorial of Bustillo y Zevallos"; and other untitled manuscripts in the Archivo General y Público.

2. Bandelier (1890:85n.) notes that relatives in Julimes of a Jumano Indian living at El Paso testified in 1732 in a witchcraft trial.

Chapter 7

1. "[E]stan enparentados unos con otros y por este se llama toda la probincia de los patarabueyes...," translated in Hammond and Rey 1929:58. An earlier use of the name Patarabueyes (but spelled "Tatarabueyes") is found in the "Declaration of Barrado, 1582," in Bolton 1916:152.
2. The Spaniards probably came to this place from the southwest. The Indians here noted that inhabitants were remote to the north and west and did not desire to go in either direction; presumably, therefore, they came to meet the Spaniards from an easterly direction. This was a disciplined tribe, showing extreme fear of the dead, and was at war with the people of the settlements. It is highly probable that a Plains Apache group is represented.
3. The Bandelier translation (1905:149–50) makes it "a river that flows between mountains." The Spanish text (Barcia 1749:34) reads, "los llevó a un río, que corría entre unos sierras...."
4. After checking the attempts made by various investigators to trace the de Vaca route, and after trying to trace it myself, I accept almost entirely the route suggested by Davenport and Wells (1919). No other route so nearly fits all the conditions, topography, rivers, vegetation, linguistic, ethnic, and cultural factors all considered.
5. Luxán notes: "We...came to a rancheria of the Patarabueyes....[P]eople from this same rancheria were taken by Mateo Gonzales, chieftain of Juan de Cubia, captain from the mines of Santa Barbara.... [Pedro]...a native of this said rancheria...was one of those taken by Matheo [*sic*] Gonzáles in the capture already mentioned" (Hammond and Rey 1929:54–56). Luxán claims that the name "Patarabueye" was made up by these same slave traders.
6. Cuchillo Parado, the "ridge barrier" or "stop," is an outstanding landmark on the Conchos River some 30 miles above La Junta. At this point the river flows through a series of high and precipitous ridges. Above is the upper valley of the Rio Conchos; below, the level and fertile valley lands of the river that extend down to La Junta.
7. This was the name the Indians gave the Spaniards for their language (Hammond and Rey 1927:16). In the Luxán diary this same group is called the "Otomoacos" (Hammond and Rey 1929:55). The Amotomancos were an outstanding Patarabueye group. Years ago Robert W. Young suggested to me that this name was quite similar to the Nahuatl form "Amoletlomanco," meaning roughly "dwellers between the yucca plants."
8. The "People of the Cows" in 1535 told Cabeza de Vaca that upstream from them he would "find nothing to eat, except a fruit they call *chacan,* that is ground between stones, and even then it could with difficulty be eaten for its dryness and pungency,—which was true" (Hodge 1907:104). It is possible that the "mushrooms" referred to by Gallegos are the "chacan" of de Vaca.
9. The usage of the term "terraced houses" in the translation is not clear. I have not seen the original Spanish text and do not know what words were actually used. "Casa terrada" as used today in northern Mexico refers not to a terraced house, but to one made of earth. This would apply much better to the La Junta house types.
10. The Conchos people on the Conchos River above La Junta were also fish eaters, as were the Tanpachoas (Mansos?) near El Paso. Regarding the latter, Luxán states:

"they fish much in the pools by means of small drag-nets" (Hammond and Rey 1929:69). This same method was probably used by the Patarabueyes, since one of the most common artifacts in La Junta archaeological sites is a small pebble, notched at both ends and often showing wear of a string or thong between the notches. Such pebbles are usually identified as "net sinkers," an identification probably correct in this instance.

11. The location of the Caguates is approximately correct for the Suma Indians, with whom they are probably to be identified.
12. This is the statement responsible for the confusion concerning Jumanos and Patarabueyes. Bolton translated it: "Having left this nation we came to another who call themselves the Jumanos, and whom the Spaniards call, for another name, Patarabueyes." Scholes (1940:275n.) quotes the original Spanish text as: "Acabados de salir de esta nación [the Tobosos], entramos en otra que se llama de los Jumanos." He points out that it would probably be better, under the circumstances, to translate this as: "Having left this nation we came to another called the Jumanos." As Scholes notes, Espejo wrote his account after his return to Santa Barbara and may have confused the "striped" Patarabueyes with the New Mexican usage of "Jumanos" to mean tattooed Indians. It is equally possible that there were Jumanos among the Patarabueyes at this time and that Espejo simply confused the two groups.

Chapter 8

1. Mendoza notes the visits of Fray García and Fray Sumesta in "Certificaciones" made at La Junta in 1684 (Mendoza, original manuscript).
2. Furthermore, the Julimes told Mendoza in 1684 that no Spaniards had been at La Junta since Sumesta's visit.
3. Indicative of the close contact the La Junta tribes had kept with the Spaniards prior to 1683 is the list of new agricultural products, including wheat, watermelons, cantaloupes, and tobacco, either of Spanish introduction or not previously noted at La Junta.

Chapter 9

1. After he returned to San Francisco de Cuellar, Trasviña Retís received letters from the priests left at La Junta asking for "peas and butter beans as there are none here now, and some garden seeds." Whether these requests were granted and these plants introduced in the La Junta region at this time is not recorded.
2. The following outline of conditions and events at La Junta to 1744, unless otherwise credited, is drawn from this account. The priests assigned to the new missions were Fray Francisco Lipiani, Fray Andrés Varo, Fray Luis Martínez [Clemente], Fray Gregorio Osorio, Fray Raymundo Graz, and Fray Antonio Aparicio. It is questionable whether this reference to the "Cumano and Zibola" refers to them at this time, or was drawn from earlier accounts of La Junta tribes.
3. In the "Letter of Don Juan de Oliván Rebolledo, Mexico, May 29, 1727" there occurs the following note: "Let his Excellency be pleased to absolve Governor Antonio Valverde from the enforcement of this judgment, and sentence him to pay fifty pesos as alms for masses for the souls of the soldiers killed in this campaign, and 150 [pesos] to help buy chalices and ornaments for the missions of La Junta de los Ríos, this being applied . . . for the souls of the deceased missionaries. He shall deliver this to the Reverend Father Vaso, their president . . . " (Hackett 1931:211–13). This would certainly suggest that the missions were in operation in 1727. Also, Orozco y Berra noted that an expedition in 1729 directed by Don José Berroteran, explored "la reunion del Rio Conchos con el del Norte or Bravo . . . ," quoted in Duro 1882. The diary of the Berroteran expedition, which I have not seen, is in the Archivo General y Público, Mexico, Historia, Vol. 52, 1, noted in Bolton 1913.

4. "Report of the Reverend Father Provincial of the Province of El Santo Evangélico to the Most Excellent Señor Viceroy... 1750," translated in Hackett 1937: 435–59 (see especially pp. 456–59). He also noted, quoting Juan de Ornedal, "It is the common opinion that each La Junta mission has at least thirty families of Indians, all domesticated and disposed to speak the Castilian language; that they produce only wheat and corn, not very abundantly ...." Ornedal had not visited La Junta himself, however.
5. Idoiaga, "Documents relating to expedition in the Junta del Rios country," quoted in Sauer 1934:67, 87; "Itinerary, diary, and autos formed by Don Fermin de Vidarre of Santiago de Mapimi, relative to his expedition to the mouth of the Conchos, 1747–1757," in the Archivo General y Público de México, Historia Vol. 52, 8; and "Pedro de Rabago y Teran, Governor of Coahuila, Diary and Report of Expedition to Junta de los Rios, 1748," also in the Archivo General y Público de México, Historia Vol. 52, 8 (noted in Bolton 1913).
6. "Las Costumbres de estos Indios vagantes,... no pueden ser más perversas, porque dominados de todas claces de vicios, y en particular de la embriaques huyen del trabajo, y simpre ambrientos y desnudos. Se robàn unos a otros cuanto pueden, ejecutande lo mismo en los demas territorios de la provincia; y dando pretidas sospechas de que cuando no se unanan con los apaches lipanes para hostilizar, les sirven de espias o les avisen el estado de nuestras poblaciones y los movimientos de las tropas para que sean menos adventurados los insultos."
7. Father Abadiano was the sole remaining missionary at San Juan at this time.
8. This reference to the Chocolomes calls for an additional note regarding this group. This is presumably the tribe elsewhere referred to as the Cholomes. The Trasviña Retís expedition in 1715 found the Cholomes living on the Rio Conchos at the pueblo of San Pedro (de Collamé), between Julimes pueblo and the pueblo of Nuestra Señora de Begoña at Cuchillo Parado. San Pedro is often referred to as a La Junta pueblo, although it is situated above Cuchillo Parado. At that time, however, most of the Cholomes lived in a "cienega" two leagues away. There were 190 persons at San Pedro at that time. They planted wheat, maize, watermelons, pumpkins, and string beans, and ate fish; they worked in the San Bartolome estates. Although described by Trasviña Retís as "most Christianized and civilized," they were often referred to in the 1680–1715 period as roving savage tribes in contrast to the more settled La Junta tribes. It appears from this Escalante reference that they had been incorporated into the La Junta pueblos by 1778, possibly as a result of Spanish colonization of the Rio Conchos above Cuchillo Parado. Sauer (1934:67) is of the opinion that the Cholomes represent a surviving Jumano group at La Junta, apparently because of their association with the Cibolas, with whom the Jumanos had previously been associated.
9. In 1937 several elderly Mexican inhabitants of the old pueblo of Pulicos, Chihuahua, were interviewed. Victorio Hernandez, then 66 years old, said that he had been born in Pulicos, and that his father Nasario Hernandez also was also born there. Alisandro Sanchez, over 70 years of age, stated that he, his father Pedro Sanchez, and his grandfather had all been born in Pulicos and had lived there all their lives. In his grandfather's time there were still Indians living there, but he did not know who they were, except that they were not Apaches. He himself helped tear down the old mission church at Pulicos. To the extent that this information can be trusted, it would seem that at least three generations of Mexican people had resided at Pulicos and that their occupation had overlapped that of the Indians.
10. "[T]he settlers of Chihuahua... suffer such poverty that they have left unprotected the Río Conchos, settled by many ranchers, who, on account of continuous robberies and murders perpetrated by the enemy, have retired up the river to La Jabonera."
11. Raht (1919) reported a Mescalero Apache legend to the effect that when they came to the Big Bend country they found it occupied by the "Cholombos" Indians, whom they killed or drove out.

12. It is probable that the 1582–1583 expeditions included Mexican Indians, guides and interpreters, and Patarabueye Indians subjected to Mexican Indian influence. The names given the Indian tribes at La Junta at that time may have been influenced by the linguistic experience of these guides. Thus, the possible Uto-Aztecan, or even Nahuatl, relationship of the term "Amotomoaco" has been commented on previously (see Chapter 7, note 7).

Chapter 10

1. Following Sayles's original survey, I have continued archaeological field work in the La Junta area in collaboration with Donald J. Lehmer. I made stratigraphic tests in one site in 1936, and in the following year completely excavated a pithouse attributed to the Concepción Focus (Kelley 1939). In 1938 the Peabody Museum-Sul Ross College Big Bend expedition excavated in a La Junta Focus component, the Shiner site (Kelley et al. 1940:73–81). Finally, in 1938 the first La Junta expedition, a cooperative undertaking of Sul Ross College and the School of American Research, utilizing labor and, in part, funds supplied by the Works Progress Administration, excavated at the Millington and Loma Alta sites near Presidio, Texas. This project was placed under my direction, but actual field supervision of the Millington site work was in the hands of Donald J. Lehmer. Preparation of the final report on these excavations has been delayed; to date only Lehmer's manuscript report summarizing the excavations and describing the architecture has been completed though I have published preliminary reports (Kelley et al. 1940:31–38; Kelley 1940:1–4).
2. This identification was made by the late George C. Vaillant (letter of February 24, 1939). Eduardo Noguera examined the same sherd and concluded that it was "early Colonial, rather than late Aztec," an identification in keeping with its association with Majolica in early Conchos Focus debris (letter of June 11, 1947). Pedro Armillas examined several other sherds from Bravo Valley components in the spring of 1947, and to our surprise identified three of these as Plumbate ware (Plate II*q*), and others as of southern Mexican affiliation (Plate II*r-t*). At his suggestion, these wares were submitted to Noguera for a check on the identification. Anna P. Shepard offered to check the "Plumbate" sherd. Noguera confirmed Aztec or possible Aztec affiliation (Plate II*r-t*). Shepard, on the other hand, promptly refuted the postulated Plumbate affiliation of the sherd inspected by her, pointing out that the temper (volcanic flour) was easily distinguishable from that of Plumbate (porphyritic rock flour), although superficially one might make the same identification as that suggested by Noguera and Armillas (Noguera, letter of June 11, 1947, and Shepard, letter of June 3, 1947). A check was made on the provenience of the specimens noted above. The ex-Plumbate specimens and two of the affinis-Aztec sherds proved to have been found in association with wares of the Chihuahua series and El Paso Polychrome sherds, and were therefore referable to the prehistoric La Junta Focus. The third affinis-Aztec sherd came from Concepción Focus debris at Loma Alta (Shafter 7:3). The situation, therefore, seems to be that wares comparable to southern Mexican wares, but not specifically identifiable, reached La Junta in prehistoric times, certainly in the thirteenth or fourteenth centuries if our Southwestern correlations are acceptable. Donald D. Brand inspected these sherds and expressed the belief that the "affinis-Aztec" specimens, however, belong with the Madera Black-on-Red series of Chihuahua, an opinion with which I concur.

Chapter 11

1. These foci were identified and their Hasinai authorship recognized by Alex D. Krieger.
2. The Nueces Focus is not well known. Sites of the focus excavated by the University of Texas (Robert T. Craig shelters in Edwards County) are stratified sites in which

the complex of artifacts associated with the Nueces Focus cannot always be separated with assurance from that of older cultures represented in the same sites.

3. The Uvalde Focus is a late complex of the Balcones Phase, and presumably of the Edwards Plateau Aspect of that phase, centered in the Nueces canyon region, but covering much of the Edwards Plateau. Diagnostic traits of the focus are thought to be Frio Flared Stem and Montell Split Stem points (Plate VIII*d, f*), and probably specialized shaft wrenches or straighteners of stone (Huskey 1935: Plate 15, No. 166, right), although these may actually belong to the Nueces Focus. The Balcones Phase itself is an early and widespread hunting and food-collecting culture of central, southern, and western Texas, characterized by many large projectile points, large blades, gouges, picks, and other core tools, primarily percussion flaked, as well as by metates and manos, and flexed inhumation in stone-protected graves.
4. In the vicinity of Waco, Texas, on the Brazos River, occur late sites with a distinctive arrowpoint type, Steiner Serrate (Plate IX). The associated complex of artifacts is not clear, but the restricted distribution of the definitive arrowpoint type suggests that the culture, tentatively termed the Trading House Focus, is to be attributed to the historic Tawakoni Indians of this area. This is reputedly the archaeological complex occurring in known historic villages of the Tawakoni. At any rate, the restricted distribution of the Trading House Focus prohibits any thought of identifying it as the culture of the Jumanos.
5. Krieger includes the plain red, brown, and yellow pottery, sand- and bone-tempered, of the Nueces, Austin, and Toyah foci in this type. Actually, it seems probable that at least two wares are represented: a thick red or brown ware, smoothed but not polished, and having sand or bone temper (Leon Plain); and a thin polished or semi-polished brown or yellow ware, often red-washed, and having a fine, compact paste, tempered with bone. The name "Doss Redware" is suggested for the latter ware, which is thought to be diagnostic of the Toyah Focus. The latter ware occasionally shows traces of scratched or shallowly engraved line designs.

Chapter 12

1. The Round Rock Focus was first described by Sayles (1935:53, Plate XIV, Table IV), and a revised account given in Kelley 1947. The Uvalde Focus was first described by Huskey (1935:108, and Plate 14, Nos. 161, 62), and apparently is the complex termed "Late Edwards Plateau" culture by Sayles (1935: Plate XII).
2. A. T. Jackson has described the pictographs of this site and illustrated several of them (Jackson 1938a:254–59, Plates CXC, CXI, CXII, and Fig. 218). An earlier paper by Julia Estill (1925) is fanciful in character, rather than factual.
3. Most of the projectile points in the site fell into easily recognizable types identified in previous work. Space does not permit detailed descriptions of artifact classes or types. The method followed in establishing the projectile point types was essentially that described by Krieger (1944).
4. For a basic description of this focus see Ray 1938. See also Kelley 1947 for a revised description.
5. The Rockport Phase (Focus) of the Texas Gulf Coast has been described by Sayles (1935:35, 40, Table 5).
6. Three superimposed alluvial formations were identified in the valley flats of the Trans-Pecos region. The deepest and oldest of these (the Neville Formation) lay directly upon the rock floor of the valley and contained the fossilized remains of mammoth and horse. Following its deposition, this formation was eroded into a "badlands" terrain. During this period of erosion, the mammoth and horse apparently disappeared and humans entered the region. A renewal of aggradation resulted in the deposition of the second formation, the Calamity Formation. Many campsites with hearths *in situ*, artifacts, and burials were incorporated in the Calamity Formation at various levels. All of these are attributed to the Pecos River Focus, a primitive gathering culture of the Balcones Phase. After the close of

Calamity deposition, renewed erosion occurred and steep-sided arroyos developed in the valley flats. During this period of erosion the Pecos River Focus disappeared from the region, and campsites attributed to the Chisos Focus, a late, partially agricultural complex of the Balcones Phase, together with burned-rock middens assigned to the Livermore Focus, appear for the first time. After a relatively short period of time, deposition was resumed and the third and last formation, termed the Kokernot, developed in the arroyo channels and over the valley flats. Sites of the Bravo Valley Aspect are found in this formation. It is thought that the Neville Formation, made up of compacted red and yellow calcareous silts, represents a period of relative humidity, probably associated with the latter part of the Wisconsin glaciation. The following period of erosion is thought to represent a time of drought, presumably immediately postglacial in age, while the humic sandy silts of the Calamity Formation represent a second period of humidity. Although Bryan and Albritton (1939) do not say so, this is perhaps subject to correlation with the "Little Pluvial" of some students. The succeeding period of erosion may represent the drought period of the late thirteenth century in the Southwest, or it may represent an even earlier and longer drought period. It is possible that the hunters of the Livermore Focus were attracted to the Davis Mountains area at this time as the result of dessication of their putative plains homeland. The Kokernot Formation is thought to represent a period of relative humidity beginning about 1300 or earlier, and it is noteworthy that farming villages of the Bravo Valley Aspect utilized the fertile and naturally irrigated flats that developed during the deposition of this formation.

7. Donald J. Lehmer (personal communication) has found Livermore Focus points in association with his Mesilla Phase, which is somewhat earlier than the El Paso Phase along the Rio Grande northward from El Paso.

Chapter 14

1. As many as ten houses were observed in one tier, but the average was much less than this. At Shafter 7:3 (Loma Alta site or San Juan Evangelista), a count based on surface indications showed an average of 4.5 houses per tier, excluding isolated houses from the count. Eight such average tiers, or 36 individual houses, would give less than nine occupants per house. If single structures were included in the count, the estimated number of occupants per room would be about fourteen persons. The latter figure seems to me a more probable estimate.
2. The name Patarabueye is given in one reference as *Tatarabueye.* Can this be a corruption of Spanish "Tatarabuelo" (great-great-grandfather), or "Tatarabuela" (great-great-grandmother)? Such a nickname might easily be applied to a people showing great respect for the aged, or using relationship terms based on age respect.
3. In view of the source, the lack of detail, and the ambiguity of these statements, they are probably of little value; nevertheless, I include them here to fill out the record.
4. Investigation of local mythology at La Junta might add considerably to this list. Thus, there is a sacred cave in the Sierra de la Cruz near La Junta, and high on the shoulder of this mountain is a modern Catholic shrine, reached by a steep, winding trail, well worn into the rock and talus of the slope. Even in the seventeenth century there were Indian reports of crosses appearing in the sky at this point, suggesting a ceremonial orientation toward it. The modern legend and the associated ceremony are of interest. According to the modern legend, the Devil used to live in the cave and spin webs out over the valley of La Junta. Maidens were caught in the webs and carried to the Devil's cave. A young priest came to La Junta many years ago and voluntarily faced the Devil in his cave. He wrestled with him there and eventually overcame him, banishing the Satanic Majesty to the depths of the cave, where he has remained ever since. One day out of the year (four days and five nights in some accounts), the Devil comes out of the cave and roams the valley. The people of La Junta spend this day (and night?) cowering in fear in their homes, keeping

their doors and windows carefully locked. With the end of this day of fear the people go out and round up the Devil. Beating on pans and yelling, they drive him slowly back toward the sierra. There, lines of fire have been built, running up the mountain to the cave. The Devil is driven between these lines of fire and back into his cave. A fire is lit before the cave entrance; once he is inside, ceremonies are performed in the shrine, and the Devil is forced to remain in the cave for another year. While this is outwardly a Catholic ceremony, it may well have been grafted onto older Indian mythology and ceremonialism. Thus, note the annual day of fear and anxiety during which evil things roam the world, the sacred cave, the use of symbolic new fire, and the fiery "antelope-trap" in which the evil is caught; all these are suggestive of Indian origin, as is perhaps the spinning of the spider web out over the valley. For a slightly different version of this ceremony and the associated myth, see Boatright 1927.

5. Nevertheless, it is my impression that the number of arrowpoints found in Patarabueye sites is much greater proportionately than is the case in Pueblo ruins. This may reflect not so much greater attention to warfare, or even hunting, but the production of arrows (or arrowpoints) as an item of trade to Plains hunters such as the Jumanos.
6. See Espejo, 1582, in Bolton 1916:174–75. The conversation was carried on by signs; hence, subtleties of meaning probably were lost.
7. That the above trade route may actually have existed, is borne out in part by the fact that trade pottery from northwestern Chihuahua occurred in quantity in the La Junta Focus levels of the Bravo Valley sites. It is curious that turquoise, maize, and cotton goods should have been obtained from the west rather than from the Piro towns farther up the Rio Grande. Actually, the Piro towns are somewhat more distant than the boundary of the *Opatería,* and the notorious Jornada del Muerto may have discouraged travel along the Rio Grande. Certainly, Rio Grande glaze ware is not found at La Junta, and the only late Pueblo IV pottery type represented in the Concepción Focus is one sherd of Jeddito Corrugated, perhaps brought back by La Junta Indians who accompanied the Rodríguez and Espejo *entradas.*
8. It is true, nevertheless, that a few sherds identified as of southern Mexican origin were found at La Junta in both La Junta and Concepción Focus levels. These may indicate direct southern contact through the Tepehuane, but they too might have come in via the Opata route. If they do represent southern contact through the Tepehuane, the contact appears to have been important.
9. See also discussion of Jumano trade. It will be recalled that implements customarily used in making arrows were not found in Toyah Focus sites, although represented in numbers at La Junta. Furthermore, arrowpoints occurred in surprisingly large numbers at La Junta. If this interpretation is correct, the Perdiz point may be a specialized product designed for the eastern trade.
10. In compiling this general list of Patarabueye culture traits, the accounts of Cabeza de Vaca and Obregón have not been used, since the former may not have referred to the Patarabueyes, and the latter shows such gross exaggeration and error that it cannot be trusted. If the de Vaca account were used, the following traits would have to be added: stone boiling in baskets or gourds; wooden tongs used in handling hot stones; houses constructed for visitors; visitors received in houses; hosts seated on floor with eyes to wall, hair pulled over their eyes, and their belongings placed in center of room. If the Obregón account were used, the following traits would be added: tortillas and tamales; bread made from mesquite; maguey; spears; weaving of cloth; "terraced" houses; gesturing, making faces, and blowing toward the sky to show respect; worshipping the sun as a god.
11. Since Pueblo villages, both modern and prehistoric, exhibit similar variability, the question apparently is not restricted to the Patarabueyes, but is of general interest.
12. This conclusion concerning the ancestry of the El Paso Phase is derived from an unpublished manuscript of Donald J. Lehmer.

Chapter 15

1. When Espejo's party stopped at the Jumano rancherias on Toyah Creek, they fished in the stream. They caught many fish, some of them so large that the Spaniards were amazed, despite the fact that Toyah Creek is a very small stream and that there were many Jumano rancherias along it. I have fished every hole along Toyah Creek, and it is my personal opinion that the existence of such large fish in this small stream can be explained only by low fishing pressure. Since the Jumano rancherias were scattered throughout the length of this stream, this may very well mean that the Jumanos did not fish at all. Notably, the notched pebbles that occur in such profusion in Patarabueye sites are lacking in Jumano sites, even when the sites lie along streams known to be rich in fish. I judge that the Jumanos had a fish taboo, in keeping with their general Plains orientation.
2. "[H]aving discussed it among themselves, they sent twelve captains in whom they most confided, to see if it were so" (Benavides, in Ayer 1916:59). "[T]hese captains, with this witness... resolved in a junta which they convoked that this witness should come to this pueblo of El Paso to ask for a minister.... " (Hackett 1931:138). "[T]hen the declarant and Don Juan Xaviata, their governor, were appointed to go at the time of their fairs to where the said strangers were ... " (Hackett 1926:271).
3. See Swanton 1942:188–89 for various descriptions of this "ceremonial" cannibalism, as practiced by the Hasinai and others.
4. This trade in bows and arrows is clearly described by de Vaca. While living with the Mariames (perhaps the Jaranames of the full historic period) of the lower Colorado or Guadalupe River, he desired to escape but was advised by his comrades, who had been with this group for some time, to wait until the time came for going to the prickly pear thickets farther down the coastal plain. At that time "people would arrive from parts farther on, bringing bows to barter and for exchange, with whom, after making our escape, we should be able to go on their return." When they reached the indicated place (a year and a half later) they found there the people of whom they had been told. "These people speak a different language, and are called Avavares. They are the same that carried bows to those with whom we formerly lived, going to traffic with them, and although they are of a different nation and tongue, they understand the other language. They arrived that day with their lodges." De Vaca himself, while among the Karankawan peoples on the coast, became a trader, carrying inland "cones and other pieces of sea-snail, conchs used for cutting, and fruit like a bean of the highest value among them, which they use as a medicine and employ in their dances and festivities. Among other matters were sea-beads." In exchange he received from the tribes of the interior, "skins, ochre with which they rub and color the face, hard canes of which to make arrows, sinews, cement and flint for the heads, and tassels of the hair of deer that by dyeing they make red." Elsewhere he notes that he "bartered with these Indians in combs... and in bows, arrows, and nets." He states that wherever he went as a trader he received fair treatment, was greeted with pleasure by the Indians, given food, and continually urged to go on such trading expeditions. It was the custom of some of these coastal plain tribes to buy wives from their enemies: "the price paid for a wife is a bow, the best that can be got, with two arrows... " See Hodge 1907:56, 61, 65, and 73.
5. This qualification is necessary. In rockshelters of the Pecos River Focus, nocked arrows with sharpened wood foreshafts and points have been found, apparently dating back to an earlier period than the introduction of stone-tipped arrows. Associated with them is a simple wooden bow. However, I am inclined to believe that even these finds date to a relatively late period, and, judging by their crudity and rarity, were not important items in the culture. Significantly, the many pictographs portraying conventionalized hunters carrying their weapons, apparently representing a highly specialized hunting cult of the Pecos River Focus, always show the use of the atlatl and darts and never the bow and arrow. Even in the same region, when human figures using the bow and arrow *are* depicted on cliff or

rockshelter walls, the style of depiction is radically different and they are usually superimposed upon older paintings.

6. The De Soto expedition in 1542 visited the province of Guasco, identifiable as one of the Hasinai towns, presumably of the Frankston Focus. Here they "found some turquoises, and shawls of cotton, which the Indians gave them to understand, by signs, were brought from the direction of the sunset" (Lewis 1907:246–47).
7. On approaching the Hasinai (Tejas) villages in 1687, Joutel "discovered three Men a Horseback, coming toward us from the Village, and being come near them, saw one dress'd after the Spanish Fashion, with a little Doublet, the Body whereof was of blue, and the Sleeves of white Fustian, as it were imbroider'd, with very straight Breeches, white worsted Stockings, Woolen Garters, a broad-brim'd flat crown'd Hat, and long Hair. We presently concluded he was a Spaniard . . ." But instead he proved to be a Hasinai Indian who had been on a journey to an Indian province in which there were Spanish priests. Going on to the village, the French found among other things "square Sword Blades, like the Spanish, on the Hilts whereof they had fastened great plumes of Feathers, and several Hawks Bells" (Joutel, in Stiles 1906:139–40). It will be recalled that two Tejas (Hasinai) Indians were at La Junta in 1683 at the time the Mendoza expedition founded missions there, and accompanied the Jumanos (and Mendoza) to the "Rio Nueces" in 1683–84. When the Jumanos left the Mendoza expedition on the Rio Nueces, the two Tejas accompanied them and presumably returned to the Hasinai towns that year or later. The Indian described here by Joutel is presumably one of these wanderers.
8. "[T]here are nuts in such abundance on this river [the "Rio Nueces," probably the Concho] that they constitute the maintenance of many nations who enjoy friendship and barter and exchange with his . . . . There are 36 nations, not counting a very great many others with which the Humanas trade and have established friendly relations . . ."

Bibliography

Manuscripts

Many of the manuscripts cited in this book are reproduced, either in the language in which they were written or in translation, in the printed works listed below. Only those manuscripts which were examined in the transcript or photostat of the original archives and which do not occur in the printed works are listed separately in this bibliography

Mendoza, Juan Antonio de
1684 Certificationes, made at La Junta while *en route* from the Jumanos, May and June. Autos Sobre los Socorros. . . , Archivo General y Público de México, Provincias Internas, Tomo 37, Expediente 4.

Revilla-Gigedo, Juan Vincente
1753 Carta del Exmo. Sr. Conde de Revilla-Gigedo con ha de 14 de Sep. y del año de 1753 para q. la Religion ponga Religiosos Misioneros en La Junta de los Ríos. Biblioteca Nacional, México, Legajo 69, Expediente 1, Folio 3. Photostatic copy in the University of New Mexico Library Archives, Albuquerque.

Tapia, Narciso
1759 Noticia de la entrada última a La Junta de los Ríos por el teniente Dn. Narciso Tapia. Biblioteca Nacional, México, Legajo 31, Expediente 5. Photostatic copy in the University of New Mexico Library Archives, Albuquerque.

Printed Materials

Albritton, Claude C., Jr., and Kirk Bryan
1939 Quaternary Stratigraphy of the Davis Mountains, Trans-Pecos, Texas. *Bulletin of the Geological Society of America,* 50:1423–74.

Appleton's New Spanish Dictionary
1925 New York.

Ayer, Mrs. Edward E., trans.
1916 *The Memorial of Fray Alonso de Benavides, 1630.* Chicago: R. R. Donnelley and Sons Co.

Bancroft, Hubert H.
1886, 1889 *History of the North Mexican States and Texas.* Vols. 15, 16. San Francisco: The History Company.

Bandelier, Adolph F.
1890 Final Report of Investigations among the Indians of the Southwestern United States. . . . *Papers of the Archaeological Institute of America, American Series,* 3. Part 1. Cambridge, Mass.: University Press.

Bandelier, Fanny
1905 *The Journey of Alvar Nuñez Cabeza de Vaca and his companions.* New York: A. S. Barnes and Co.

Barcía Carballido y Zuñiga, Don Andrés Gonzalez de
1749 *Historiadores primitivos de las Indias Occidentales.* Tomo I, Madrid.

Boatright, Mody C.
1927 The Devil's Grotto. *Texas and Southwestern Lore.* Publications of the Texas Folk-Lore Society, 4:102–6.

Bolton, Herbert E.
1911 The Jumano Indians in Texas, 1650–1771. *The Quarterly of the Texas State Historical Association,* 15(1):66–84.
1912 The Spanish Occupation of Texas, 1519–1690. *Southwestern Historical Quarterly,* 16:1–26.
1913 Guide to Materials for the History of the United States in the Principal Archives of Mexico. Washington, D.C.: Carnegie Institution. Publication 163.
1916 *Spanish Exploration in the Southwest, 1542–1706.* New York: Charles Scribner's Sons.
1924 The Location of La Salle's Colony on the Gulf of Mexico. *Southwestern Historical Quarterly,* 27:171–89. Reprinted from the *Mississippi Historical Review,* 2:165–82.

Casey, Clifford B.
1933 The Trans-Pecos in Texas History. *West Texas Historical and Scientific Society Publications,* 5:10–15.

Cox, Isaac Joslin
1905 *The Journeys of René Robert Cavelier Sieur de La Salle.* New York: Allerton Book Co.

Davenport, H., and J. K. Wells
1919 The First Europeans in Texas, 1528–1536. *Southwestern Historical Quarterly,* 22(2, 3):111–42, 205–59.

Duro, Cesáreo Fernández
1882 *Don Diego de Penalosa y Su Descubrimiento del Reino de Quivira.* Madrid.

Estill, Julia
1925 Indian Pictographs Near Lange's Mill, Gillespie County. *Publications of the Texas Folk-Lore Society,* 4:103–14.

Hackett, Charles W.
1923, 1926, 1937 *Historical Documents Relating to New Mexico, Nueva Vizcaya, and Approaches Thereto, to 1773.* Vols. 1, 2, and 3. Washington, D.C.: Carnegie Institution. Collected by Adolph F. A. Bandelier and Fanny Bandelier.
1931, 1934 *Pichardo's Treatise on the Limits of Louisiana and Texas.* Vols. 1, 2. Austin: University of Texas Press.

Hallenbeck, Cleve
1940 *Alvar Nuñez Cabeza de Vaca: The Journey and Route of the First European to Cross the Continent of North American, 1534–1536.* Glendale, Calif.: Arthur H. Clark Co.

Hammond, George P., and Agapito Rey
1927 The Gallegos Relation of the Rodriguez Expedition to New Mexico. *Historical Society of New Mexico Publications in History,* 4. Sante Fe, N.M.: El Palacio Press.
1928 *Obregón's History of 16th Century Exploration in Western America.* Los Angeles: The Quivira Society.
1929 *Expedition into New Mexico Made by Antonio de Espejo, 1528–1583, As Revealed in the Journal of Diego Peréz de Luxán, a Member of the Party.* Los Angeles: The Quivira Society.

Hatcher, Mattie Austin
1927 Descriptions of the Tejas or Asinai Indians, 1691–1772. *The Quarterly of the Texas State Historical Association,* 30(3):206–18.
1932 The Expedition of Don Domingo Teran de los Rios into Texas. *Preliminary Studies of the Texas Catholic Historical Society,* 2(1). Austin, Tex.: St. Edward's University. Distributed under the auspices of the Texas Knights of Columbus Historical Commission.

Haury, Emil W.
1936a The Mogollon Culture of Southwestern New Mexico. *Medallion Papers,* 20. Gila Pueblo.
1936b Some Southwestern Pottery Types, Series IV. *Medallion Papers,* 20. Gila Pueblo.

Hodge, Frederick Webb
1907 The Narrative of Alvar Nuñez Cabeza de Vaca. *Spanish Explorers in the Southern United States, 1528–1543,* pp. 3–126. New York: Barnes and Noble.
1911 The Jumano Indians. *Proceedings of the American Antiquarian Society,* n.s. 20:249–68.

Holden, W. C.
1938 Blue Mountain Rock Shelter. *Bulletin of the Texas Archaeological and Paleontological Society,* 10:208–21.

Hughes, Anne E.
1935 *The Beginnings of Spanish Settlement in the El Paso District.* El Paso, Tex.: Press of the El Paso Public Schools. Reprinted from the *University of California Publications in History,* 1(3). Berkeley: University of California Press.

Huskey, Vane
1935 An Archaeological Survey of the Nueces Canyon of Texas. *Bulletin of the Texas Archaeological and Paleontological Society,* 7:105–14.

Jackson, A. T.
1938a Picture Writing of the Texas Indians. The University of Texas Publications, 3809. Anthropological Papers, 2.
1938b The Fall Creek Sites. *Annual Report of WPA and The University of Texas Archaeological Research, Lake Buchanan, 1936*–1937. The University of Texas Publications, 3802. Anthropological Papers, 3(1).

Kelley, J. Charles
1933 Report on Archaeological Field Work in the Madera Valley Area. *West Texas Historical and Scientific Society Publications,* 5:53–59.
1937 The Route of Antonio de Espejo . . . Its Relation to West Texas Archaeology. *West Texas Historical and Scientific Society Publications,* 5:7–25.
1939 Archaeological Notes on the Excavation of a Pithouse Near Presidio, Texas. *El Palacio,* 46(10):221:34.
1940 Recent Field Work in Texas: (1) Presidio. *Texas Archaeological News,* 2:1–4.
1947 The Cultural Affiliations and Chronological Position of the Clear Fork Focus. *American Antiquity,* 13(2):97–109.

Kelley, J. Charles, T. N. Campbell, and D. J. Lehmer
1940 The Association of Archaeological Materials with Geological Deposits in the Big Bend Region of Texas. *West Texas Historical and Scientific Society Publications,* 10.

Krieger, Alex D.
1944 The Typological Concept. *American Antiquity,* 9(3):271–88.
1946 Culture Complexes and Chronology in Northern Texas. The University of Texas Publications, 4640.

Lewis, Theodore H.
1907 The Narrative of the Expedition of Hernando de Soto by the Gentleman of Elvas. *Spanish Explorers in the Southern United States, 1528–1543,* pp. 127–272. New York: Barnes and Noble.

Margry, Pierre
1875– 1886 *Découvertes et établissements Des Français dans l'Ouest et dans le Sud de l'Amérique Septentrionale (1614–1754).* Vol. 3, *Recherche des Bouches du Mississipi...* Paris: Imprimerie de D. Jouaust.

Mera, H. P.
1938 Reconnaissance and Excavation in Southeastern New Mexico. Memoirs of the American Anthropological Association, 51.

Portillo, Esteban L.
1886 *Apuntes para la Historia Antigua de Coahuila y Texas.* Saltillo, Mexico.

Raht, Carlysle Graham
1919 *The Romance of the Davis Mountains and Big Bend Country: A History.* El Paso, Tex.: Raht Books Co.

Ray, Cyrus N.
1929 A Differentiation of the Prehistoric Cultures of the Abilene Section. *Bulletin of the Texas Archaeological and Paleontological Society,* 1:7–22.
1935 The Pottery Complex Artifacts of the Abilene Region. *Bulletin of the Texas Archaeological and Paleontological Society,* 7:70–88.
1938 The Clear Fork Culture Complex. *Bulletin of the Texas Archaeological and Paleontological Society,* 10:193–207.

Ray, Cyrus N., and E. B. Sayles
1941 An Agreement on Abilene Region Terminology. *Bulletin of the Texas Archaeological and Paleontological Society,* 13:175–176.

Reindorp, Reginald C.
1938 The Founding of Missions at La Junta de los Rios. *Supplementary Studies of the Texas Catholic Historical Society,* 1(1). Reprinted from *Mid-America,* n.s. 9(2).

Sauer, Carl
1932 The Road to Cibola. *Ibero-Americana,* 3. Berkeley: University of California Press.
1934 The Distribution of Aboriginal Tribes and Languages in Northwestern Mexico. *Ibero-Americana,* 5. Berkeley: University of California Press.

Sayles, E. B.
1935 An Archaeological Survey of Texas. *Medallion Papers,* 17. Gila Pueblo.
1936 An Archaeological Survey of Chihuahua, Mexico. *Medallion Papers,* 22. Gila Pueblo.

Scholes, F. V., and H. P. Mera
1940 Some Aspects of the Jumano Problem. *Contributions to American Anthropology and History,* 34. Washington, D. C.: Carnegie Institution. Publication 523.

Smith, Victor J.
1928 Spanish Exploration in the Big Bend of Texas. *West Texas Historical and Scientific Society Publications,* 2.

Stiles, Henry Reed
1906 *Joutel's Journal of La Salle's Last Voyage.* Albany.

Swanton, John R.
1942 Source Material on the History and Ethnology of the Caddo Indians. *Bureau of American Ethnology, Bulletin,* 132.

Vetancurt, Fray Agustín de
1698 *Teatro Mexicano: Descripción Breve de los Sucesos Ejemplares, Históricos y Religiosos del Nuevo Mundo de las Indias. Crónica de la Provincia del Santo Evangélio de Mexico.* Facsimile of the original document printed in 1971 by Editorial Porrúa, Mexico.

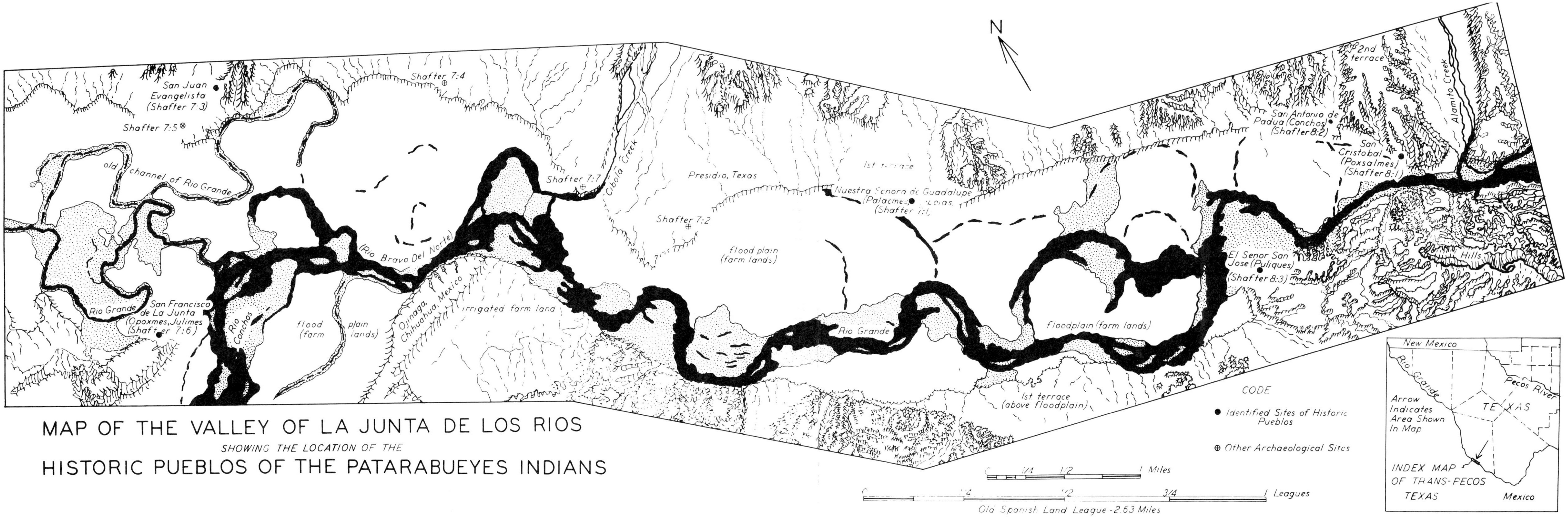

MAP OF THE VALLEY OF LA JUNTA DE LOS RIOS
SHOWING THE LOCATION OF THE
HISTORIC PUEBLOS OF THE PATARABUEYES INDIANS